Rapid Ps

KT-103-225

Rapid Psychiatry

Clare Oakley
Specialty Registrar in Forensic Psychiatry
Birmingham and Solihull Mental Health Foundation Trust

Amit Malik
Consultant Psychiatrist
Hampshire Partnership NHS Trust

Second Edition

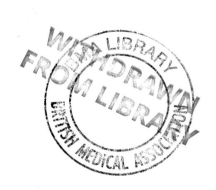

WILEY-BLACKWELL

A John Wiley & Sons, Ltd., Publication

This edition first published 2010, © 2010 by C. Oakley and A. Malik

Previous editions: 2004

Blackwell Publishing was acquired by John Wiley & Sons in February 2007. Blackwell's publishing programme has been merged with Wiley's global Scientific, Technical and Medical business to form Wiley-Blackwell.

Registered office: John Wiley & Sons Ltd, The Atrium, Southern Gate, Chichester, West Sussex, PO19 8SQ, UK

Editorial offices: 9600 Garsington Road, Oxford, OX4 2DQ, UK
The Atrium, Southern Gate, Chichester, West Sussex, PO19 8SQ, UK
111 River Street, Hoboken, NJ 07030-5774, USA

For details of our global editorial offices, for customer services and for information about how to apply for permission to reuse the copyright material in this book please see our website at www.wiley.com/wiley-blackwell.

Library of Congress Cataloging-in-Publication Data

Oakley, Clare.
Rapid psychiatry / Clare Oakley, Amit Malik. – 2nd ed.
p. ; cm. – (Rapid series)
ISBN 978-1-4051-9557-7
1. Brief psychotherapy–Handbooks, manuals, etc. I. Malik, Amit. II. Title.
III. Series: Rapid series.
[DNLM: 1. Mental Disorders–Handbooks. 2. Psychiatry–methods–Handbooks.
WM 34 O11r 2010]
RC480.55.H53 2010
616.89'14–dc22

2010015125

ISBN: 9781405195577

A catalogue record for this book is available from the British Library.

Set in 7.5/9.5pt Frutiger-Light by Thomson Digital, Noida, India.

Printed and bound in Malaysia by Vivar Printing Sdn Bhd

1   2010

Contents

Neuropsychiatry

Child and Adolescent Psychiatry

Old Age Psychiatry

Psychiatry of Learning Disability

Forensic Psychiatry

Psychotherapy

Psychopharmacology

Appendices

Glossary

Preface

It has been an absolute joy and challenge to complete this book for undergraduate medical students. *Rapid Psychiatry* is set out in 11 different sections. In addition to the introduction, differential diagnosis, psychopharmacology and the appendices which cover topics that are relevant across the range of patient groups and clinical settings, the book contains sections on the main areas of specialism within psychiatry. Within most sections, the chapters are arranged in alphabetical order except for the introduction and appendices chapter which do not lend themselves well to such an arrangement. We hope that this book will make the undergraduate experience more enjoyable for all medical students and that many more will decide to choose psychiatry as their future career.

Acknowledgements

We are both grateful to Allison Hibbert, Alice Goodwin and Frances Dear whose excellent original work provided the inspiration for this second edition. We would also like to thank Dr Helen Smith for her invaluable contributions regarding the Scottish mental health legislation. This book would not have been possible without our own teachers and the authors of many reference textbooks and scientific papers whose wisdom has been sieved in the subsequent pages. Whilst the format of the book did not lend itself to referencing every expert and publication, we thank them all. The team at Wiley-Blackwell have supported us throughout this process, from Joan Marsh, who first introduced us to the publication house, to Ben Townsend, whose enthusiasm convinced us to take on this project, and finally to Laura Murphy, whose patience and support have guided this book through its many revisions. And finally we thank our families for their patience and support through our hours of writing and revising the text.

List of Abbreviations

5-HIAA	5-hydroxyindoleacetic acid
5-HT	5-hydroxytryptamine (serotonin)
AA	Alcoholics Anonymous
ABC	Airway, breathing, circulation (basic life support)
ABG	Arterial blood gases
ACE	Angiotensin-converting enzyme
ADHD	Attention deficit hyperactivity disorder
AMHP	Approved mental health practitioner
AMP	Approved medical practitioner
APP	Amyloid precursor protein
AV	Atrioventricular
AWI	Adults with Incapacity (Scotland) Act 2000
BMI	Body Mass Index
BNF	*British National Formulary*
BP	Blood pressure
Ca	Calcium
CBT	Cognitive-behavioural therapy
CJD	CreutzfeldtJakob disease
CMHT	Community Mental Health Team
CNS	Central nervous system
CPN	Community psychiatric nurse
CRP	C-reactive protein
CSF	Cerebrospinal fluid
CT	Computed tomography
CTO	Compulsory Treatment Order
CVA	Cerebrovascular accident/stroke
CXR	Chest X-ray
DKA	Diabetic ketoacidosis
DSM	*Diagnostic and Statistical Manual of Mental Disorders* (US diagnostic guidelines)
DZ	Dizygotic
ECG	Electrocardiogram
ECT	Electroconvulsive therapy
EDC	Emergency Detention Certificate
EEG	Electroencephalogram
EMDR	Eye Movement Desensitisation and Reprocessing
EPSE	Extrapyramidal side effect
ESR	Erythrocyte sedimentation rate
EtOH	Ethanol (alcohol)
FBC	Full blood count
FTA	Fluorescent treponemal antibody test

GABA	γ-aminobutyric acid
GAD	Generalised anxiety disorder
GCS	Glasgow Coma Scale
GGT	γ-glutamyl transferase
GI	Gastrointestinal
GP	General practitioner
GPI	General paresis of the insane
HIV	Human immunodeficiency virus
HR	Heart rate
IBS	Irritable bowel syndrome
ICD	*International Classification of Diseases* (WHO diagnostic guidelines)
ICP	Intracranial pressure
IM	Intramuscular
IQ	Intelligence quotient
ITU	Intensive therapy unit
IV	Intravenous
LD	Learning disability
LFT	Liver function test
LP	Lumbar puncture
LSD	Lysergic acid diethylamide
MAOI	Monoamine oxidase inhibitor
MDT	Multidisciplinary team
MHA	Mental Health Act (1983)
MHO	Mental health officer
MI	Myocardial infarction
MMR	Measles, mumps and rubella
MMSE	Mini mental state examination
MRI	Magnetic resonance imaging
MSE	Mental state examination
MSU	Midstream urine
MZ	Monozygotic
NA	Noradrenaline (norepinephrine)
NSAID	Non-steroidal anti-inflammatory drug
OCD	Obsessive-compulsive disorder
OT	Occupational therapy
PD	Personality disorder
PTSD	Post-traumatic stress disorder
RC	Responsible clinician
RMO	Responsible medical officer
SOAD	Second opinion approved doctor
SSRI	Selective serotonin reuptake inhibitor
STDC	Short-Term Detention Certficate
TCA	Tricyclic antidepressant
TFT	Thyroid function test

TIA	Transient ischaemic attack
TMS	Transcranial magnetic stimulation
TPHA	*Treponema pallidum* haemagglutination assay (test for syphilis)
U&E	Urea and electrolytes
UTI	Urinary tract infection
VDRL	Venereal Diseases Reference Laboratory
WHO	World Health Organization

Introduction to Psychiatry

Summary

The following are the broad headings of a standard psychiatric assessment, which are discussed in detail later in the chapter. Special considerations for specific patient groups (children, older people, etc.) are discussed at the beginning of relevant chapters.

Psychiatric history

- Patient's personal details
- Presenting complaint
- History of presenting complaint
- Past psychiatric history
- Past medical history
- Drug history
- Family history
- Personal history:
  - Childhood
  - School
  - Occupations
  - Psychosexual history
  - Alcohol and substance use
  - Forensic history
  - Social situation
- Premorbid personality

Mental state examination

- Appearance and behaviour
- Speech
- Mood
- Thought
- Perception
- Cognition
- Insight

Signs and symptoms

Affect is the observable behaviour of a subjectively experienced emotion. It is variable over time (in comparison to mood which is a pervasive and sustained emotional state). Affect may be:

- *blunted* – lack of appropriate emotional response to events
- *flat* – absence of expression of affect
- *inappropriate* – affect is inappropriate to the thought or speech it accompanies
- *labile* – rapid changes in affect.

Anxiety is a feeling of apprehension, uneasiness or tension. It is accompanied by somatic sensations including sweating, palpitations and shortness of breath. Anxiety may be free-floating (pervasive) or related to a specific fear (phobic).

Compulsions are stereotyped acts, recognised as excessive, unreasonable or exaggerated. If the patient tries to resist doing them, there is a sense of mounting tension that can be immediately relieved by yielding to the compulsion. Often involve:

- cleaning
- checking
- counting
- hoarding.

Delusions are abnormal beliefs which are held with absolute certainty. They are based on incorrect inferences about external reality and are firmly held despite proof or evidence to the contrary. They are not beliefs which can be understood as part of their cultural or religious background. The beliefs are usually but not always false – for example, the patient's spouse may actually be having an affair. It is the abnormal thought processes that define a delusion, not whether the belief is true.
Delusions may be classified as primary or secondary.

- **Primary delusions** do not have any identifiable connection with previous events and are a direct result of the psychopathology. Types of primary delusion are:
  o *autochthonous* – 'out of the blue', fully formed beliefs
  o *delusional memory* – arising from a memory
  o *delusional mood* – arising from a period of anticipatory anxiety and the sense that something was about to happen
  o *delusional perception* – an abnormal belief arising from a normal perception (e.g. the traffic lights turn red and the patient realizes that is a sign they are the next Messiah).
- **Secondary delusions** arise out of another primary psychiatric symptom (e.g. low mood) and are understandable in the context. They are a product of an attempt to understand the primary morbid experience.

Common types of delusion include the following.

- *Persecutory* – being conspired against, attacked or persecuted.
- *Grandiose* – inflated self-worth, special powers or abilities, relationships with important and special people, having a mission.
- *Reference* – events have a particular and unusual significance for the patient, they are being referred to on television and in the newspapers.
- *Delusions of control (passivity phenomena)* – being controlled by an external agent:
  o emotions
  o impulses
  o actions
  o somatic passivity (bodily sensations).

- *Thought interference (passivity phenomena)* – thoughts are controlled by an external agency:
  o thought withdrawal
  o thought broadcast
  o thought insertion.
- *Misidentification* – certain individuals are not who they appear to be. Familiar people have been replaced with outwardly identical strangers (Capgras syndrome) or strangers are really familiar people (Fregoli syndrome).
- *Guilt* – believe they deserve punishment.
- *Nihilistic* – they have died or no longer exist or that the world has ended.
- *Hypochondriacal* – believe they have a serious physical illness.
- *Jealousy* – partner is being unfaithful (Othello syndrome).
- *Love* – another person, usually of higher status, is deeply in love with them (de Clerambault syndrome).
- *Infestation* – their skin is infested with multiple insects or parasites (Ekbom syndrome).

Delusions may be mood congruent, e.g. grandiose in elated mood states and nihilistic in depressed mood states, or mood incongruent, e.g. grandiose in depressed states.

Depressed mood is the core feature of a depressive illness. Patients describe a pervasive unhappiness, being unable to feel happy, hopelessness, helplessness and negative thoughts about themselves, the world and the future. Other features of a depressive illness are discussed in the relevant section.

Elevated mood is the core feature of a manic illness. Patients describe feeling very happy, being positive about everything, feeling indestructible, feeling more creative, being able to think more quickly and achieve more tasks than usual. Other features of a manic illness are discussed in the relevant section.

Formal thought disorder refers to an abnormality of the form of thought.

- *Circumstantiality* – irrelevant and unnecessary details are incorporated into the thinking, meaning that the goal of the thought is reached very slowly.
- *Flight of ideas* – accelerated thoughts with abrupt changes to related thoughts. The connections between the thoughts may be based, for example, on puns, rhyming words or alliteration.
- *Loosening of associations* – lack of meaningful connection between thoughts:
  o derailment – thought derails onto a subsidiary thought
  o drivelling – disordered mixture of the constituent parts of one thought
  o fusion – two or more unrelated concepts are brought together
  o omission – part of a thought is omitted
  o substitution – a thought is substituted by a subsidiary thought.
- *Neologism* – a new word constructed by the patient or an existing word used in a new way.

Hallucinations are perceptions without the corresponding external object. The subjective experience is a normal perception in that sensory modality (i.e. voices sound like 'real' voices). A true hallucination will be perceived in external space and be outside conscious control.

- *Auditory:*
  o second-person – voices directly addressing the patient (e.g. 'you are useless')
  o third-person – two or more voices discussing the patient (e.g. 'he's very powerful')
  o thought echo – voices echo thoughts before or after they happen
  o running commentary – voices comment on action (e.g. 'he's going out of the door now').

Signs and symptoms (continued)

- *Visual* – e.g. small figures seen in delirium.
- *Olfactory* – usually an unpleasant smell.
- *Gustatory* – commonly a feeling that something tastes differently and this is often interpreted as being the result of poisoning.
- *Somatic* – e.g. sensation of insects under skin or movement of joints.

Illusions are false perceptions of a real external stimulus. There are three types:

- *affect* – during heightened emotion (e.g. when walking alone on a dark night, seeing a shadow as an attacker)
- *completion* – 'filling in' of presumed missing parts of an image (e.g. optical illusions)
- *pareidolic* – produced when experiencing a poorly defined stimulus (e.g. seeing faces in the clouds).

Obsessions may be persistent thoughts, images, doubts or impulses. They are acknowledged as originating in the mind and are repetitive and intrusive. The patient tries to resist them. The obsessions cause distress and interfere with functioning. Common content includes:

- contamination
- bodily fears
- aggression
- orderliness/symmetry.

Overvalued ideas are an unreasonable and sustained intense preoccupation. It is not of delusional intensity (the person can acknowledge that it is possible the belief may not be true). The ideas can be understood but are incorrect and can come to dominate the person's life.

Pseudo-hallucinations are a form of imagery arising in the subjective inner space of the mind and not perceived as part of the external world. They do not have the same quality as normal perceptions. They can occur in any sensory modality but are most commonly auditory.

Psychiatric history
Patient's personal details

- Name
- Age
- Gender
- Marital status
- Occupation
- Religion/ethnic group

Presenting complaint

- Document this in the patient's own words.
- Document how long the patient has had the problem, e.g. 'feeling low for the last few months'.
- Use open-ended questions to elicit these, e.g. 'Can you tell me about the problems that brought you here?'.
- Let the patient speak uninterrupted for the first few minutes before continuing questioning.

History of presenting complaint

- When did the problem start?
- Has it changed over time? If so, how?
- Were there any precipitating events, e.g. bereavement, divorce?
- Any psychological/drug treatments for the current problem? If so, did they help?
- Screen for any other problems. All patients should be asked about suicidal ideation, depression, anxiety, obsessional behaviour and psychosis.

Past psychiatric history

- Have they seen a psychiatrist before?
- Have they been treated by their GP for any mental health problems?
- Have they been treated in hospital before?
- Were they detained under mental health legislation?
- Are there any previous risk behaviours (deliberate self-harm, violence, aggression, etc.) related to their previous mental health problems?

Past medical history

- Enquiry regarding any significant illnesses, operations or accidents.

Drug history

- Do they take any regular medication?
- What medication have they taken previously for their mental health and was it effective?

Family history

- Is there a family history of mental illness?
- Collect information about parents, siblings and other significant relatives.
- Enquire about age, occupation, social circumstances and quality of the relationship with the patient.
- Make a genogram (family tree) of the information.

Personal history

- *Childhood* – birth history (difficulties, prematurity); developmental milestones, delay in particular; description of early childhood; family and home atmosphere.

Psychiatric history (continued)

- *School* – leaving age; any truancy or school refusal, bullying; relationships with peers, teachers; exams taken and qualifications, further education.
- *Occupations* – list all jobs and duration of employment, reasons for leaving and any periods of unemployment.
- *Psychosexual history* – current relationship if any, sexual orientation, any sexual difficulties, first sexual experience, any sexual abuse, past significant relationships – reasons why they ended.
- *Alcohol and substance use* – alcohol, tobacco and illicit drugs; record amount, e.g. units of alcohol per week; current and previous use; patterns of use; symptoms/signs of dependency and withdrawal; associated problems, e.g. financial difficulties.
- *Forensic history* – record all offences whether convicted or not (especially note violent crimes, sexual crimes and persistent offending).
- *Social situation* – type of housing, who else is at home; financial circumstances including income, benefits, debts; social support – friends, relatives, social services.

Premorbid personality

- Difficult to assess in a short interview. Focus on consistent patterns of behaviour throughout life. This part should include an account from an informant, as no individual can objectively describe their own personality. Useful questions include 'How would you describe yourself when well?' and 'How would others describe you?'.
- *Areas to include* – attitudes to others in relationships; attitudes to self; predominant mood; leisure activities and interests; reaction to stress, coping mechanisms.

Mental state examination
Appearance and behaviour

- *Dress, self-care* – e.g. bright colours and flamboyant clothing may be seen in mania, self-neglect in depression.
- *Behaviour during the interview* – restlessness, tearfulness, eye contact, irritability, appropriateness, distractibility.
- *Psychomotor* – poverty of movement, stereotypes, rituals, other abnormal movements.
- *Level of rapport* established during interview.

Speech

- *Rate* – slow/retarded, pressured/uninterruptible.
- *Tone* – normal, monotone or excessive intonation.
- *Volume* – whisper, quiet, loud.
- *Content* – monosyllabic, spontaneous or only in answer to questions.
- Dysphasia or dysarthria.

Mood

- *Objectively* – your impression – depressed, elated, euthymic, blunted or flattened, anxious.
- *Subjectively* – how the patient reports prevailing mood – depressed, elated.

It is usual to also record any thoughts of self-harm or suicide here.

Thought

- Formal thought disorder
- Passivity of thought
- Overvalued ideas
- Obsessions, compulsions, ruminations
- Beck's cognitive triad – negative views of self, the world and the future
- Delusions

Perception

- *Sensory distortions* – increase in sound or colour sensitivity.
- *Illusions* – a misinterpretation of normal stimuli.
- *Hallucinations* – false perceptions in the absence of any stimulus.

Cognition

- Consciousness, orientation, concentration, attention.
- Memory: the Mini-Mental State Examination (MMSE) is a widely used bedside test which screens for cognitive problems. It includes elements such as orientation, attention, short-term memory, naming objects and following verbal and written commands. A score out of 30 is obtained, with a score of less than 25 being suggestive of dementia. The MMSE does not assess frontal lobe function and this will need to be considered by other tests.

Insight

- Does the patient believe they are unwell?
- What do they think is causing it?
- Are they willing to accept help?

Mental state examination (continued)
Formulation

- *Summary* – aim to give a very short précis of the relevant points of the case. Include the following: patient's demographic details, relevant background information, chronological presenting symptoms, relevant mental state examination findings.
- *Differential diagnosis* – it is important not to forget organic causes, as these can be easily reversible and require different management. Simple blood tests are important, for example:
  - o anaemia causes fatigue which is also found in depression
  - o thyroid abnormalities can mimic depression or mania
  - o calcium abnormalities can cause depression
  - o renal failure and liver failure can cause delirium.
- *Aetiology* – consider biological, psychological and social issues (use the grid below to fit these together).

Factors	Biological	Psychological	Social
Predisposing (what made this problem likely?)			
Precipitating (what triggered it?)			
Perpetuating (why is it still going on?)			

- Management plan:
  - o need for history from other informants
  - o physical examination
  - o blood tests and other investigations
  - o risk assessment
  - o psychological assessment
  - o OT assessment
  - o consideration of social circumstances and accommodation
  - o psychological therapies
  - o medication
  - o involvement of MDT
  - o use of relevant legislation.
- Prognosis.

Classification systems for mental disorders
International classification of diseases (ICD-10)

- International classification system
- Published by the World Health Organization (WHO)
- Covers all physical and mental illnesses and disorders
- Psychiatric disorders covered in Chapter V of ICD-10
- Categorical classification of diagnosis
- Single axis of diagnosis using the concept of co-morbidities
- Used more commonly in clinical settings within the UK

Diagnostic and statistical manual of mental disorders (DSM-IV)

- National classification system used in the United States of America
- Developed by the American Psychiatric Association
- Exclusively covers psychiatric disorders
- Classification characterised by operational diagnosis
- Multiaxial system of diagnosis which includes:
  - Axis I – Clinical syndromes
  - Axis II – Developmental disorders and personality disorders
  - Axis III – General medical conditions
  - Axis IV – Psychosocial and environmental problems
  - Axis V – Global assessment of function
- Used more commonly in the USA but less so in the UK

Assessment of suicide risk

All patients being evaluated psychiatrically should be assessed for suicide risk. Never be afraid to ask about suicide – simply by asking, you will not increase the likelihood of a patient committing suicide and remember that identifying a suicide risk can prevent a patient committing suicide. Make sure the setting is calm, quiet and private. Establish a good rapport – use a calm, understanding and sympathetic approach.

Suicide risk is increased by a sense of hopelessness, the presence of psychiatric and medical illnesses, the presence of recurring suicidal thoughts, recent stressful events (e.g. loss of job or bereavement) and previous attempts at suicide. The risk is increased if the suicidal thoughts have led to formulating a plan as to how to go about it. A lack of social support also contributes to an increased risk, as does a lack of strong 'preventing' factors such as religious belief or children to look after. These factors must be asked about in order to assess the patient's suicide risk. Below are some suggested questions that could be used for assessing suicide risk.

Eliciting a sense of hopelessness

- Do you still get pleasure out of life?
- How do you feel about the future?
- Does life seem worth living?
- Are you able to face each day?
- Do you ever wish you would not wake up?
- Do you find there are things to live for? Tell me about them.

Suicidal thoughts

- Have you ever thought of ending it all?
- Are you able to resist the thoughts?
- How do you feel about these thoughts?
- Have you ever thought about methods of suicide?
- Have you ever made any plans?
- Have you started to put these plans into action?

Previous attempts

- Have you ever tried anything before? Can you tell me about it?

Social support

- Have you ever told anyone before about how you feel?
- Do you have someone to confide in, close family or friends?
- Who do you live with – do you have company at home?

Identifying stressors that increase the risk

- Is there something in particular that is making you feel worse? Can you tell me about it?

Preventing factors

- What might prevent you from carrying out any plans?

Health problems

- Do you know if you are suffering from any mental health problems?
- Do you have any other health problems that are bothering you?

Deliberate self-harm

DEFINITION Intentional self-inflicted injury/harm without a fatal outcome.

AETIOLOGY

- 'Cry for help' – to obtain relief, to escape a situation, to seek attention or to make someone feel guilty
- Impulsivity
- Poor coping strategies
- Self-punishment
- Failed suicide attempt

ASSOCIATIONS/RISK FACTORS

- Single/divorced
- Lower social classes
- Previous history of child abuse
- Unemployment
- Recent stressful event, e.g. loss of loved one, being in trouble with the law
- Borderline personality disorder
- Depression
- Substance misuse

EPIDEMIOLOGY Incidence of 3 per 1000 in UK but this is probably an underestimate. More prevalent in lower social classes and those living in crowded urban areas. More common in women and those under 35 years.

HISTORY This should focus on obtaining a clear account of events and intentions in order to undertake a risk assessment of future risk of self-harm and suicide.

Indicators of serious suicidal intent

- A planned and premeditated attempt, e.g. 'I have been collecting the packets of paracetamol for weeks, I have been buying a packet a week with my shopping'.
- Attempt carried out in isolation and precautions taken to avoid discovery, e.g. 'I locked my door so no one could get in'.
- Final acts in anticipation of death, e.g. 'I had written suicide notes and posted them to all my friends and family'.
- Violent, dangerous methods, e.g. 'I knew that if I tried to cut the veins in my neck, it would be more effective than slitting my wrists'.
- Person thought the act would be final and irreversible, e.g. 'I thought that 10 paracetamol would be enough to kill me'
- They did not seek help after the act, e.g. 'I am angry that my flatmate came home unexpectedly and called the ambulance'.
- Person regrets surviving the attempt, e.g. 'I wish I'd made a better job of it'.
- Numerous previous attempts, e.g. 'This is the third time I have tried to kill myself; I am a failure, I can't even do that right'.

EXAMINATION Mental state examination may reveal a psychiatric disorder, which is of crucial importance in determining future risk and should be suitably managed once identified.

INVESTIGATIONS None specifically.

MANAGEMENT

- Treat as medically appropriate.
- Full assessment – assess risk and need for hospital admission. Use MHA if necessary.
- Treatment of underlying psychiatric disorders.

Deliberate self-harm (continued)

- A small minority of patients will present frequently with deliberate self-harm without suicidal intent. An individualised management plan should be agreed that does not reward maladaptive behaviours but provides appropriate support.

COMPLICATIONS   Repeated self-harm, unintentional suicide, suicide.

PROGNOSIS   One percent will commit suicide within the next 2 years. This means that this group is at 100 times greater risk of suicide than the general population. Hence the need for a psychiatric assessment following deliberate-self-harm.

Suicide

DEFINITION   Intentional self-inflicted death. Not all suicide attempts result in death. It can be difficult to distinguish between those that were intended to be fatal and those that were acts of deliberate self-harm.

AETIOLOGY

- *Psychiatric disorders* (90% of those who commit suicide have a psychiatric disorder):
  o depression (15% of patients commit suicide)
  o schizophrenia (10% of patients commit suicide)
  o substance misuse
  o personality disorder
  o anorexia nervosa.
- *Medical disorders* – chronic pain and cancer patients.
- *Biochemical abnormalities* – studies of CSF and brain show reduced 5-HIAA.
- *Social factors* – loss of shared values and reduced social support.

ASSOCIATIONS/RISK FACTORS

- Previous deliberate self-harm
- *Age* – young men and elderly are at higher risk
- *Sex* – M > F
- Loss events (e.g. bereavement)
- Unemployment
- Living alone
- Single, divorced or widowed

EPIDEMIOLOGY   Annual incidence in England and Wales is approximately 1 in 10,000; rates vary between countries. Highest rates in the elderly, although rates rising in young men. It is more common in men than women.

PREVENTION

- Individual level
  o Detection of people at risk of psychiatric disorders
  o Effective management of psychiatric disorders
- Population level
  o Reduce ease (e.g. smaller packets of paracetamol)
  o Provide support services (e.g. Samaritans)
  o Reduce stressors (e.g. reduce unemployment)
  o Reduce stigma of mental health (e.g mental health campaigns with MIND)

Multidisciplinary team

This is the team of professionals who are responsible for the long-term care of the patient. The advantage of working in this type of team is that all the patients' needs can be properly addressed and comprehensive care provided. Psychiatric patients benefit greatly from psychological and social input in addition to their medical care. Multidisciplinary teams (MDTs) operate on wards, in day hospitals and in the community. All members of the team will attend ward rounds and meetings concerning the patient.

Members of the MDT

- Psychiatrists
  - o Assessment and diagnosis of mental illnesses
  - o Decision making and liaison regarding management
  - o Recommendations for detention under the Mental Health Act if required
  - o Prescribing and monitoring of medication
  - o Management of physical health problems
- Psychiatric nurse
  - o Monitoring and observations of inpatients
  - o Administration of medication
  - o Involved in decision making about leave arrangements for detained patients
- Community psychiatric nurse
  - o Monitoring of outpatients in the community
  - o Visiting patients at home regularly to assess mental state and review progress
  - o Giving depot injections
- Social worker
  - o Involving the patient's family with their care
  - o Finding appropriate accommodation
  - o Assisting with other social issues, such as benefits
  - o Assessments of vulnerable adults and child protection issues
- Occupational therapist
  - o Helping people reach their maximum level of function and independence in all aspects of daily life
  - o Assessment of activities of daily living
  - o Developing skills to assist with attending courses or returning to employment
- Clinical psychologist
  - o Assessment of patients' suitability for psychological treatment
  - o Psychological assessments including intelligence tests and personality assessments
  - o Psychological treatment of patients, for example cognitive behavioural therapy

Patient advocates are not members of the MDT but help the patients express their opinions and any concerns they may have. They may attend meetings with the patient to make requests on behalf of the patient.

Ethical issues

The practice of psychiatry requires detailed consideration of important ethical and legal issues. This is essential as psychiatric care often requires making decisions on behalf of patients or detaining and treating patients against their will. As this over-rides a patient's right to make their own decisions, it is crucial that this occurs within an ethical and legal framework. The relevant mental health legislation is discussed later in this section. The ethical principles are outlined below.

Respect for autonomy

Patients should be treated as rational autonomous agents who are allowed to make decisions regarding their treatments. From this principle, other requirements follow, including informed consent and confidentiality. Respect for a patient's autonomy assumes that they have the capacity to make rational choices. However, capacity can be impaired in both physical and mental illnesses. The assessment of capacity is an important skill for all doctors.

Beneficence

This is the requirement to do good and promote well-being. This should be the guiding principle of doctors' interactions with patients.

Non-maleficence

'First, do no harm.' This is difficult to separate from the principle of beneficence, as in almost all therapeutic decisions a judgement is made about the balance of benefits against the potential harm. A common example is the prescription of medication; consideration is given to the intended outcome of taking the medication and the side effects that may be experienced and the medication will only be prescribed if the potential benefits outweigh the potential harm. These judgements should be a collaboration between the patient and doctor, such that the patient's autonomy regarding decision making is optimised.

Justice

This principle refers to distributive justice, which is concerned with the fair distribution of resources between individuals. The British NHS was founded on the principle of equal access to treatment which is free at the point of need. The reality of limited resources leads to difficult decision making and establishing of priorities.

Mental Capacity Act

Mental capacity is the ability to make a decision. The Mental Capacity Act became law in 2005 and provides the legal framework for:

- people who lack capacity to make decisions for themselves
- people who have capacity and want to make provisions for when they might lose capacity in the future.

Principles of mental capacity

1. Mental capacity is decision and time specific, i.e. it is incorrect to say that an individual lacks mental capacity generally; rather, one should state that an individual does/not lack capacity to make a specific decision at a specific time.
2. An individual must always be presumed to have capacity unless proven otherwise.
3. An assessor, whilst making an assessment of mental capacity, must do everything possible to enhance an individual's capacity to make the decision in question.
4. Every adult has a right to make their own decisions (even unwise ones!) if they have mental capacity to do so.
5. In cases of individuals lacking capacity, those making decisions on their behalf must do so in their best interest.

Assessment of mental capacity

Assessment of capacity is a two-stage process and must be undertaken keeping the above principles in mind.

- *Stage I* Does the person have an impairment of mind or brain?
- *Stage II* If so, does the impairment mean that the person is unable to make the decision in question at the time it needs to be made?

To assess whether an individual is able to make the decision, one must assess their ability to understand, retain and weigh up information relevant to the decision and then communicate their decision by any means.

Lasting power of attorney (LPA)

An LPA gives the chosen person (attorney or donee) authority to make decisions that are as valid as ones made by the person (donor) themselves. An LPA can cover:

1. property and affairs decisions
2. welfare decisions.

Court of Protection

This is the special court set up to deal with decision making for adults who may lack capacity to make specific decisions for themselves.

Advance decision

An advance decision enables someone aged 18 or over, while still capable, to refuse specified medical treatment for a time in the future, when they may lack capacity to consent to or refuse that treatment.

Adults With Incapacity (Scotland) Act 2000

The Adults With Incapacity (Scotland) Act 2000 (AWI) is the equivalent legislation in Scotland to the Mental Capacity Act in England and Wales. The AWI has a number of principles with which the decisions regarding the adult should be made:

1. Beneficence
2. Minimum intervention
3. Consideration of the wishes of the adult
4. Consultation with relevant others
5. Encouraging the adult to exercise residual capacity

The assessment of capacity is the same as in England and a number of features are very similar. The AWI allows for the person to appoint a Power of Attorney which will continue if the person becomes incapable. There is also a Welfare Power of Attorney to make decisions regarding personal welfare.

An application is made to the Sheriff Court for an intervention order or a guardianship order. The intervention order is designed for one-off decisions; if there are ongoing concerns about the person's capacity then a guardianship order would be applied for. Both of the interventions require three reports: two from doctors and one from a social worker.

The AWI can authorise medical treatment, financial interventions and the adult taking part in research. The AWI does not allow for the use of force or detention in hospital. If the adult is being kept in hospital against their will then the Mental Health (Care and Treatment) (Scotland) Act 2003 should be considered.

Mental health legislation
Mental health legislation varies in different countries
The legislation for Scotland is detailed later but initially the Mental Health Act 1983 of England and Wales is considered. This legislation was amended in 2007. It applies to any patient with a mental disorder who needs to be detained in hospital but some sections (37, 47, 48, 49 and 41) are more common in the practice of forensic psychiatry due to their relation to the courts.

Mental Health Act 1983 of England and Wales

Criteria for detention

- In order to be detained under the Mental Health Act (MHA), a person must be determined to be suffering from a **mental disorder**. There is no definition in the legislation of 'mental disorder' other than that it is a disorder or disability of the mind. However, detention solely on the basis of dependence on alcohol or drugs is not permitted.
- It is also necessary to decide that the **nature** or **degree** of the mental disorder warrants detention in hospital (for assessment or treatment depending on the section used).
- It must be necessary for the **health** or **safety** of the patient or the **protection of others** that the patient be detained in hospital.
- For detention under section 3 or related treatment sections. **appropriate medical treatment** must be available. This is defined as *'medical treatment, the purpose of which is to alleviate, or prevent a worsening of, the disorder or one or more of its symptoms or manifestations'*.

Professionals involved

The following professionals may be involved in the process of detention under the Mental Health Act, depending on the section under which the patient is detained.

- Section 12(2) approved doctor, who has been certified to have special expertise in mental health. Their role is to provide a medical recommendation for detention.
- In most cases a second medical recommendation is required and this must be independent of the first and ideally someone who has prior knowledge of the patient (patient's GP). If this is not possible, a second section 12(2) approved doctor's recommendation is usually used.
- Approved mental health practitioner (AMHP) is a role that was previously carried out by approved social workers but since the 2007 amendments to the MHA, can be taken on by other mental health professionals. AMHPs have received specific training relating to the application of the MHA. In relation to civil sections (section 2, 3, 4 and Community Treatment Orders), AHMPs make the application for detention to the hospital based on the medical recommendations and other relevant information.
- The responsible clinician (RC) is the approved clinician in charge of the patient's care. It replaces the previous term of responsible medical officer (RMO). At the time of writing, RCs are all psychiatrists but the 2007 amendments allow other mental health professionals to take up this role after special training.

Mental health review tribunals

- Patients may appeal their detention under the MHA by applying for a tribunal.
- The tribunal consists of an independent panel of a psychiatrist (usually a consultant), a lawyer and a lay person.
- They may decide to discharge the patient from hospital if they are satisfied that the criteria for detention are not met.

Section 5(2)

- Requires a recommendation by the RC or their nominated deputy who may be a doctor or an approved clinician (it is often the on-call psychiatric trainee).
- Maximum duration 72 hours during which a full MHA assessment should take place.

Section 2

- Requires two medical recommendations (as described above) and the recommendation of an AMHP.
- Maximum duration 28 days.
- Is for assessment of a mental disorder (and treatment if required).

Section 3

- Requires two medical recommendations and the recommendation of an AMHP.
- Initial duration is 6 months and can be extended by a further 6 months and then for periods of 1 year at a time.
- Is for treatment of a mental disorder.

Sections 47, 48 and 49

- These involve the transfer of patients from prison to hospital for assessment and treatment of mental disorders.
- Section 48 is used for remand prisoners (awaiting trial).
- Section 47 is used for sentenced prisoners.
- Section 49 is a restriction that is used in combination with section 47 or 48. It is imposed to protect the public from serious harm. Under this restriction, any leave of absence, transfer between hospitals or discharge must be sanctioned by the Ministry of Justice.

Sections 37 and 41

- Section 37 is a hospital order and is similar to a section 3. It is imposed by a court instead of a prison sentence on the basis of two medical recommendations.
- Section 41 is a restriction order that may also be imposed by the court in conjunction with a Section 37 if it is deemed necessary to protect the public from serious harm.
- Section 37/41 patients can only be discharged:
  - o by a tribunal or
  - o by the RC seeking the Ministry of Justice's approval.
- Once patients subject to section 37/41 are discharged, they will have to comply with conditions of their discharge, such as taking medication, or they will be recalled to hospital.

Community treatment orders

- Supervised community treatment was introduced in the 2007 amendments to the MHA.
- Community Treatment Orders may be used for patients who have been detained under section 3 or 37.
- They allow patients to live in the community whilst still being subject to the powers of the MHA for the purpose of receiving medical treatment and they can be recalled to hospital.

Other powers

- *Section 136* – police can detain people whom they believe to be mentally disordered in a public place to a place of safety for up to 72 hours.
- *Section 135* – magistrate can issue a warrant allowing entry to private premises to search for and remove patients thought to need urgent medical attention.
- *Section 5(4)* – nurses' holding power for inpatients that lasts for up to 6 hours.

Mental health legislation (continued)

- *Section 4* – emergency section of up to 72 hours requiring only one medical recommendation and application by an AHMP.
- *Section 17 leave* – leave from the hospital for patients detained under the MHA that must be approved by the RC.
- *Section 58* – this is concerned with consent to treatment and 3 months after medication is first administered, the patient must consent to it or the treatment plan must be agreed by a second opinion approved doctor (SOAD).
- *Section 117 aftercare* – patients who have been detained under section 3 or equivalent are entitled to free aftercare arrangements, including appropriate accommodation.

Mental Health (Care and Treatment) (Scotland) Act 2003

Criteria for detention

- The patient should have (or be suspected of having) a mental disorder. This is defined in the act as a mental illness, personality disorder or learning disability.
- Medical treatment would be likely to alleviate the symptoms or prevent worsening of the mental disorder.
- If the patient was not given the treatment, there would be a significant risk to the health, safety or welfare of the patient or to the safety of others.
- The patient has significantly impaired decision-making abilities about the treatment of their mental disorder.
- There is no other option but for the patient to receive this treatment (least restrictive option).

Exclusions for detention

A person cannot be defined as having a mental disorder for any of the following reasons:

o Sexual orientation
o Sexual deviancy
o Trans-sexualism/transvetism
o Dependence on or the using of drugs or alcohol
o Behaviour that causes alarm or distress to another person
o Acting as no prudent person would act

Professionals involved

- An approved medical practitioner (AMP) is a psychiatrist approved under section 22 of the Mental Health (Care and Treatment) (Scotland) Act 2003 as having special experience and expertise in the diagnosis and treatment of mental disorders. This is usually a ST4 or above.
- A responsible medical officer (RMO) is the consultant psychiatrist in charge of the patient's care.
- Mental health officers (MHOs) are social workers trained in dealing with people with mental health problems. The MHO is consulted to assess if the patient requires detention under the Mental Health Act.
- The patient has a 'named person' whom the clinical team must consult about the treatment and detention of the patient. This is usually a relative but can be anybody nominated by the patient.
- Mental health tribunals are the same as in England and Wales.

Emergency detention certificate (EDC/Section 36)

- Any doctor with General Medical Council full registration can complete this but the person should be reviewed as soon as possible by an AMP.

- Can last for 72 hours.
- Only allows for detention in hospital and assessment, NOT treatment.
- Should be with MHO consent but in emergencies can be completed without.
- There is no right of appeal against this section.

Short-term detention certficate (STDC/Section 44)

- Is implemented by an AMP and MHO.
- Lasts for 28 days.
- Allows for treatment as well as assessment.
- Can be appealed against with application to the mental health tribunal.
- Has to be declared for travel purposes (e.g. visas to visit the USA).
- Should be used in preference to the EDC for the detention of patients.

Compulsory treatment orders (CTOs/Section 63)

- This section is granted by the mental health tribunal.
- There are two recommendations made to the tribunal, by the RMO and another doctor, usually an AMP. The MHO is also consulted and should be in agreement.
- Is initially for a period of 6 months; this can be extended for 6 months and then renewed annually if required.
- It can be appealed against to the mental health tribunal.
- CTOs can be hospital based or community based, which allows for compulsory treatment in the community.

Other powers

- As with the English Mental Health Act, there are other powers available to the police and nursing staff holding powers.
- Patients can be moved from the courts and prisons for assessment/treatment of their mental health.
- These transfers are completed under the Criminal Procedures (Scotland) Act 1995 as amended by the Mental Health (Care and Treatment) (Scotland) Act 2003.
- The sections used depend on where in the legal process the patients are; for more information, see the Mental Health (Care and Treatment) (Scotland) Act 2003 Code of Practice, all three volumes of which are available on the Scottish government website.
- The Mental Health Act forms are also available online.

Differential Diagnosis

The anxious patient
Symptoms
Emotions: anxiety, tension, irritability.

Cognitions: exaggerated fears and worries.

Behaviour: avoidance of feared situation, checking, seeking reassurance.

Somatic features: tight chest, hyperventilation, palpitations, decreased appetite, nausea, tremor, aches and pains, insomnia, frequent desire to pass urine.

Differential diagnosis
Psychiatric

- Generalized anxiety disorder
- Panic disorder
- Phobias
- Obsessive compulsive disorder (OCD)
- Post-traumatic stress disorder (PTSD)
- Acute stress reaction
- Depression
- Substance misuse – especially withdrawal symptoms
- Personality disorder
- Dementia

Medical

- Hypoglycaemia
- Hyperthyroidism
- Phaeochromocytoma
- Delirium

Management

- Psychiatric history and mental state examination.
- Exclude medical disorders – blood pressure, glucose, full blood count, thyroid function tests, etc.
- Acute anxiety may be relieved by anxiolytics, e.g. benzodiazepines, but for short courses only as patients may become dependent on them if they are used in the long term.
- Certain antidepressants can be used for treatment of anxiety disorders, even if the patient is not depressed, e.g. citalopram for panic disorder and venlafaxine for generalized anxiety disorder.
- Cognitive-behavioural therapy.

The depressed patient
Symptoms
Core features: persistent low mood, anhedonia, anergia.

Cognitive features: decreased concentration and attention, low self-esteem, bleak and pessimistic views of the future, feelings of guilt or worthlessness, ideas of self-harm or suicide.

Somatic features: poor sleep, early morning wakening, decreased appetite leading to weight loss, decreased libido, constipation, amenorrhoea, diurnal variation of mood, psychomotor retardation.

Differential diagnosis
Psychiatric

- Depression
- Severe depression with psychotic symptoms
- Bipolar affective disorder
- Anxiety disorder
- PTSD
- Schizophrenia
- Schizoaffective disorder
- Dementia
- Substance misuse (chronic alcohol misuse)
- Personality disorder

Medical

- Hypothyroidism
- Cushing syndrome
- Hypercalcaemia (malignancy)
- Infections (HIV, syphilis)
- Multiple sclerosis
- Parkinson disease
- Medication (sedatives, anticonvulsants, β-blockers)

Others
Bereavement.

Management

- Psychiatric history and mental state examination (assess for suicidal ideation and manic and psychotic features).
- Exclude medical cause for depression.
- Antidepressants.
- Cognitive-behavioural therapy.

The elated patient

Symptoms

Main features: elevation of mood, overactivity, pressure of speech, disinhibition.

Other features: irritability, flight of ideas, distractibility, grandiose ideas, decreased sleep, impaired judgement, irresponsibility, decreased appetite.

Differential diagnosis

Psychiatric

- Hypomania
- Mania
- Mania with psychotic symptoms
- Schizoaffective disorder
- Schizophrenia
- Acute intoxication with cocaine or amphetamines
- Acute and transient psychotic disorder

Medical

- Brain disorders affecting the frontal lobes (e.g. space-occupying lesion, dementia, HIV infection, syphilis)
- Alcohol withdrawal
- Corticosteroids
- Anabolic androgenic steroids
- Hyperthyroidism

Management

- Psychiatric history and mental state examination.
- During the interview maintain a calm, non-confrontational manner. Manic patients may become aggressive or violent in response to even minor irritations.
- Exclude other medical causes.
- Antipsychotics and benzodiazepines are used in an acute episode.
- Lithium and other mood stabilisers are used as prophylaxis in bipolar affective disorder.
- ECT can be used in severe cases of mania resistant to other treatment.

The hallucinating patient
Symptoms
Auditory, visual, somatic, olfactory or gustatory hallucinations. Auditory and somatic are more likely in psychiatric disorders, while visual and olfactory suggest an organic disorder.

Differential diagnosis
Psychiatric

- Schizophrenia
- Schizoaffective disorder
- Delusional disorder
- Mania with psychotic symptoms
- Severe depression with psychotic symptoms
- Acute and transient psychotic disorder
- Alcohol and drug misuse, e.g. hallucinogenic drugs – LSD, 'magic mushrooms'
- Delirium tremens

Medical

- Temporal lobe epilepsy
- Space-occupying lesion
- Delirium
- Metabolic disturbances, e.g. liver failure
- Infection – encephalitis
- Head injury

Management

- Psychiatric history and mental state examination (including risk assessment).
- Exclude organic disorders.
- Antipsychotic drugs for psychosis.
- Consideration should be given to admitting the patient to hospital.

The patient with obsessions/compulsions
Symptoms
Obsessions are unwanted, distressing thoughts or images that enter the patient's mind even though they try to resist them. The thoughts are recognised as the patient's own.

Compulsions are acts performed to ease the anxiety caused by obsessions and become repetitive and are recognised as senseless.

Differential diagnosis

- OCD
- Anankastic personality disorder
- Depression
- Schizophrenia
- Anorexia nervosa
- Phobic disorders
- Tourette's syndrome

Management

- Psychiatric history and mental state examination.
- Consider if there are any other symptoms that might suggest depression or psychosis.
- Antidepressants – clomipramine and SSRIs have the greatest efficacy.
- Cognitive-behavioural therapy.

The unresponsive patient
Symptoms

- Alert with eye movements only.
- Mutism (absent speech).
- Absent movements.
- Decreased attention span for environmental stimuli.
- Speech may be present but there may be amnesia for personal identity and history.

Differential diagnosis
Psychiatric

- Schizophrenia (catatonic state)
- Depression (depressive stupor)
- Neuroleptic malignant syndrome
- Dissociative disorders

Medical

- Hypoglycaemia
- Delirium
- Encephalitis
- Parkinson disease
- Cerebrovascular accident
- Acute intoxication, e.g. alcohol, solvents

Management

- ABC.
- Exclude life-threatening brain pathology.
- Check vital observations – BP, pulse, GCS.
- Initially obtain brief history from an informant (? known psychiatric illness, medication, illicit substances; is the patient deaf and/or blind? what language does the patient speak?).
- Perform complete physical examination.
- Perform investigations guided by the history and examination.
- Ensure that the patient is adequately hydrated – IV fluids.
- Once life-threatening brain injury has been excluded, obtain a full history from an informant, obtain old notes and attempt MMSE on the patient.
- Admit the patient; further management will depend on the underlying aetiology.

General Adult Psychiatry

Anxiety disorders – agoraphobia

DEFINITION Anxiety associated with places or situations from which escape may be difficult, e.g. crowds and public places.

AETIOLOGY Family and twin studies suggest that genetic factors are relevant. Onset of agoraphobia often follows a precipitating event, which may be a panic attack, which leads to avoidance. It can occur following a major life event in someone with dependent personality traits.

ASSOCIATIONS/RISK FACTORS It is strongly associated with panic and ICD-10 classifies the disorder into agoraphobia either with or without panic disorder.

EPIDEMIOLOGY F > M. Average age of onset is late twenties.

HISTORY Consistent and marked fear of:

- crowds
- public places
- travelling alone
- being away from home

Anxiety symptoms occur in the feared environment or in anticipation of it:

- Palpitations
- Sweating
- Shaking
- Dry mouth
- Difficulty breathing
- Chest pain
- Nausea
- Dizziness
- Hot flushes
- Fear of losing control
- Fear of dying

Avoidance of these situations is the prominent feature. The patient may feel better if accompanied by someone else.

EXAMINATION Normal unless in that situation. May have a panic attack if exposed.

INVESTIGATIONS FBC, U + Es, LFTs, Ca, TFTs.

MANAGEMENT Exposure therapy, gradually increasing, e.g. walking increasing distances from home each day. CBT.

COMPLICATIONS Isolation. Secondary depression. May misuse alcohol or illicit substances to cope with feared environment.

PROGNOSIS Fluctuating course. Condition may be severe and the person housebound.

Anxiety disorders – generalised anxiety disorder

DEFINITION   Generalised and persistent anxiety, not restricted to, or predominating in, any particular circumstances (free-floating).

AETIOLOGY

- Genetic predisposition
- Current stress
- Life events

ASSOCIATIONS/RISK FACTORS   Childhood experiences characterised by separations, demands for high achievement and excessive conformity.

EPIDEMIOLOGY   Lifetime prevalence is 5%. F > M. Onset is in adolescence to early adulthood.

HISTORY   The symptoms should be present most days for at least several weeks at a time. These symptoms should involve elements of:

- apprehension (worries about future misfortunes, feeling on edge, difficulty concentrating)
- motor tension (restlessness, fidgeting, tension headaches, trembling)
- autonomic overactivity (lightheadedness, sweating, tachycardia or tachypnoea, dizziness, dry mouth, epigastric discomfort).

EXAMINATION   Tachycardia and tachypnoea.

INVESTIGATIONS   FBC, U + Es, LFTs, Ca, TFTs.

MANAGEMENT

- Anxiety management:
  o psychoeducation
  o distraction techniques
  o cognitive control
  o breathing/relaxation techniques
- Benzodiazepines may be useful in the short term.
- SSRIs or venlafaxine are useful.

COMPLICATIONS   Half will develop a depressive illness. May misuse alcohol or illicit substances to cope with anxiety.

PROGNOSIS   Course may be chronic, worse at times of stress. Poor prognosis is associated with longer duration of illness, co-morbid psychiatric disorder and poor premorbid personality.

Anxiety disorders – social phobia

DEFINITION   Persistent fear of social situations that may lead to scrutiny, criticism or embarrassment (e.g. eating, drinking, speaking in public).

AETIOLOGY   There is evidence from family studies of a genetic component.

ASSOCIATIONS/RISK FACTORS   More likely in those with lifelong sensitivity to critiscism and avoidant personality disorder.

EPIDEMIOLOGY   F > M. Onset gradual from late adolescence.

HISTORY   Situational anxiety in social groups: parties, meetings, classrooms. There is marked avoidance of these situations. There will be anxiety symptoms and blushing, trembling, fear of vomiting and urgency/fear of micturition.

EXAMINATION   Normal unless exposed to social situation. Then blushing, shaking, restless, avoids eye contact. Fear of scrutiny/humiliation. Fear of vomiting/fainting.

MANAGEMENT   Graded exposure and desensitisation. CBT. SSRIs.

COMPLICATIONS   Social phobia may be secondary to a depressive illness when social performance declines. Secondary alcohol and substance misuse is common.

PROGNOSIS   Generally present for life.

Anxiety disorders – specific phobia

DEFINITION   Persistent fear of a specific object or situation, out of proportion to the threat of the situation. The fear is recognised as excessive, but cannot be reasoned away.

AETIOLOGY   There is evidence for a familial pattern of phobias. Classical conditioning suggests that phobias arise as a result of a negative experience with the object or situation. Phobias may also develop by modelling (i.e. watching parents).

ASSOCIATIONS/RISK FACTORS   Biological vulnerability to anxiety. Hypervigilant individuals more at risk.

EPIDEMIOLOGY   F > M. Blood/needle/injury phobia F = M. Twelve-month prevalence is approximately 10% of the population. Onset usually in childhood, but may vary.

HISTORY   Symptoms of anxiety and panic when exposed to feared stimulus. Fear and avoidance of specific objects or situations. Types of phobias include:

- animals
- blood/injury
- heights
- illness.

Anxiety symptoms include:

- sweating
- trembling
- dry mouth
- nausea
- difficulty breathing
- choking sensation
- chill/hot flushes.

Most phobias cause tachycardia but blood/injury phobia causes an initial tachycardia followed by vasovagal bradycardia and hypotension. This may cause nausea and fainting.

EXAMINATION   Normal unless exposed to feared stimulus. When exposed, sweating, restless, panic, distracted, fearful.

MANAGEMENT   Systematic desensitisation: relaxation therapy paired with graded exposure. Use of benzodiazepines in the short term may allow the patient to engage more easily in systematic desensitisation.

COMPLICATIONS   Disruption of normal daily life if the phobic stimulus is something that must be routinely encountered.

PROGNOSIS   Good. Exposure therapy is often successful. Most phobias do not interfere with normal life if the stimulus can be easily avoided.

Chronic fatigue syndrome

DEFINITION A term used to describe an idiopathic syndrome characterised principally by the occurrence of months of extreme disabling fatigue coupled with other somatic symptoms such as muscle pain and resulting in impairment of function.

AETIOLOGY Unknown and controversial.

ASSOCIATIONS/RISK FACTORS

- High prevalence of lifetime psychiatric illness
  o Mild depression
  o Anxiety
  o Somatisation
- Infection – patients often give a history of acute symptoms of viral infection
- May develop after Epstein–Barr virus infection (glandular fever)
- Some evidence for precipitating life events
- Associated with other medically unexplained syndromes including IBS and fibromyalgia

EPIDEMIOLOGY Prevalence is approximately 1% of the population. F > M.

HISTORY Physical and mental fatigue must have been present for 6 months in order to make the diagnosis. Common symptoms include:

- lack of energy
- exhaustion after minimal effort
- muscular weakness
- poor concentration and memory
- lack of endurance
- sleep disturbance
- dizziness
- inability to relax
- irritability
- aches and pains
- headaches
- dyspepsia.

EXAMINATION May be co-morbid features of anxiety and depression. All patients presenting with fatigue need a full physical examination.

INVESTIGATIONS Although the syndrome is idiopathic, investigations should be performed to exclude other pathology. FBC, ESR/CRP, U&E, glucose, TFT, antinuclear antibody tests should be routinely considered in all patients presenting with fatigue.

MANAGEMENT

- Offer appropriate explanations, reassurance and hope.
- For mild cases, patients can be advised to build up endurance gradually, starting with a manageable level and increasing a little each day.
- Give advice about sleeping patterns – encourage regular sleep pattern, avoid excessive rest/sudden changes in activity. Avoid drinking stimulants, e.g. caffeine, especially before bedtime.
- For more severe cases, patients may benefit from CBT based on a more formal exercise programme, and assessment using all the members of the MDT, e.g. physiotherapist, OT, psychologist.
- Antidepressant treatment will help for co-morbid depression or anxiety.

COMPLICATIONS Interrupts social functioning, e.g. relationship problems, unemployment.

Chronic fatigue syndrome (continued)

PROGNOSIS Depends on severity. If mild symptoms, management in general practice may have a good outcome. Most have recovered by 2 years. However, if symptoms are severe and require hospital admission, the prognosis is poorer and tends to follow a chronic course.

Dissociative disorders

DEFINITION A general definition is physical or mental symptoms that occur in the absence of a physical disorder to explain them. However, DSM-IV and ICD-10 differ in their classification of the symptoms. In DSM-IV, dissociative disorders refer to mental symptoms and conversion disorders refer to physical symptoms. ICD-10 refers to both types of symptoms as dissociative disorders, and the terms dissociative and conversion disorder may be used interchangeably. The ICD-10 practice is used in the lists below.

AETIOLOGY Used to be called hysteria. Psychodynamic theories suggest that dissociative symptoms are caused by the repression of unconscious intrapsychic conflict and the conversion of the resulting anxiety into a physical symptom. This results in the relief of emotional conflict (primary gain) and the advantages of assuming the sick role (secondary gain). Preliminary functional brain imaging suggests identifiable changes which are different from those of people who are feigning illness.

ASSOCIATIONS/RISK FACTORS There are convincing associations in time with stressful life events, insoluble problems and disturbed relationships. It is associated with childhood abuse and other traumatic experiences.

EPIDEMIOLOGY Rare disorder. Thought to be more common in women and younger adults.

HISTORY The patients often show less distress than would be expected of someone with their symptoms, sometimes called 'belle indifférence'. However, they often show exaggerated emotional reactions to other things.

The condition must be distinguished from malingering, in which the patient consciously and deliberately feigns illness in order to avoid a situation, e.g. prison.

Types of dissociative state include the following:

- *Dissociative amnesia* – core feature is a patchy loss of memory, usually of recent traumatic events.
- *Dissociative fugue* – same features as dissociative amnesia with an apparently purposeful journey away from home. A new identity may be assumed.
- *Dissociative pseudo-dementia* – the patient shows abnormality of intelligence, suggesting dementia, but answers questions wrongly in a way that suggests they have the correct answer in mind.
- *Dissociative stupor* – motionless and mute, but they are aware of their surroundings.
- *Dissociative disorders of movement and sensation* – the symptoms often resemble the patient's idea of a physical disorder. The core feature is loss of function which does not appear to be under voluntary control.

EXAMINATION There must be *no evidence* of a physical disease that can explain the symptoms of this disorder.

INVESTIGATIONS Exclude physical cause for the symptoms. This may be difficult.

MANAGEMENT

- Resolution is usually spontaneous and may be helped by supportive therapy aimed at increasing insight and stress management and coping skills.
- Reassure the patient that serious physical illness is excluded.
- The patient should not be confronted but should be allowed to discard the symptoms without losing face.
- Minimise the advantages of the sick role.

COMPLICATIONS These conditions may become chronic due to the secondary gain (disorder confers some advantage to the patient, e.g. excused from usual responsibilities).

PROGNOSIS Usually excellent but chronicity is possible, as above.

Eating disorders – assessment

In addition to the standard psychiatric assessment, the following questions should be asked when an eating disorder is suspected.

Weight

o What is your current weight?
o How often do you weigh yourself?
o What has your weight been in the past (highs and lows)?

Eating

o Tell me about what you normally eat on a typical day, say yesterday.
o Are you dieting at the moment?
o Do you ever binge? What do you eat and what do you do afterwards? How do you feel during a binge?
o Do you think about food frequently?
o Do you eat out with friends?
o Do you like shopping for food/cooking?
o Have you ever used any methods of losing weight other than dieting?
o What exercise do you do?
o Have you tried slimming pills?
o Do you take laxatives/diuretics?
o Do you ever make yourself sick after eating?

Body image

o Do you feel fat?
o Are you dissatisfied with particular parts of your body?
o What do you think about your body shape?
o What would your ideal weight be?
o Do you think you need to lose weight?
o If somebody said you needed to put on weight, how would that make you feel?

Physical problems associated with weight loss

o Are your periods regular?
o Are you interested in sex?
o Do you feel tired and weak?
o Do you suffer from dizziness?

Eating disorders – anorexia nervosa

DEFINITION   Eating disorder characterised by deliberate weight loss resulting in a weight 15% below expected or a BMI <17.5, with secondary endocrine and metabolic disturbances.

AETIOLOGY

- Genetic (MZ > DZ concordance, increased risk if family history)
- Dysfunction of 5-HT neurotransmitter system
- Sociocultural view that thinness is attractive
- Family relationships, e.g. over-involved parents
- Personality, e.g. perfectionism, low self-esteem, obsessive traits

ASSOCIATIONS/RISK FACTORS   It is associated with certain occupations, e.g. ballet and modelling. Co-morbid depression, substance misuse and personality disorder are common.

EPIDEMIOLOGY   95% are female. Peak age of onset is 15–19 years. Prevalence is approximately 1–2 per 1000 women. There is a higher prevalence in higher socio-economic classes and Western Caucasians.

HISTORY

- Weight loss induced by diet restriction and one or more of:
  o Self-induced vomiting
  o Excessive exercise
  o Appetite suppressants or diuretics
  o Laxatives
- Morbid fear of fatness
- Body image distortion
- Loss of libido
- Fatigue
- Amenorrhoea
- Obsessional thoughts and rituals

EXAMINATION   It is essential to exclude a medical cause for the weight loss. A patient with anorexia may:

- be gaunt and emaciated
- be dehydrated
- have proximal myopathy
- have cold extremities
- have bradycardia and hypotension
- have fine lanugo hair
- exhibit peripheral oedema
- have parotid gland enlargement and erosion of tooth enamel (secondary to vomiting).

They may be low in mood. There will be a preoccupation with food and overvalued ideas about weight and appearance. Insight is usually poor.

INVESTIGATIONS   FBC, U&E, LFT, amylase, lipids, glucose, TFTs, Ca, magnesium, phosphate. ECG due to electrolyte abnormalities. Bone scan may be indicated if osteoporosis is suspected.

MANAGEMENT

- Correct medical complications (may require admission to medical ward)
- Psychiatric admission if very low weight or suicide risk
- Refeeding via nasogastric tube if necessary
- Negotiate dietary aims

Eating disorders – anorexia nervosa (continued)

- Psychoeducation and supportive psychotherapy
- Monitor muscle power, BP, biochemistry, weight
- CBT
- Family therapy
- SSRIs

COMPLICATIONS

- Osteoporosis
- Cardiac arrhythmias
- Renal failure
- Pancreatitis
- Hepatitis
- Seizures
- Peripheral neuropathies
- Suicide

PROGNOSIS Variable. Some patients recover after a single episode, some relapse and some run a chronic deteriorating course over many years. Half of patients will have no eating disorder at long-term follow-up. There is a substantial mortality of 10% due to complications of the eating disorder and suicide. Poor outcome is associated with older age of onset, long duration of illness, lower weight at presentation and poor childhood social adjustment.

Eating disorders – bulimia nervosa

DEFINITION   Eating disorder characterised by uncontrolled binge eating with vomiting/laxative abuse. There is a preoccupation with body weight and shape.

AETIOLOGY   Those with bulimia are more likely to have a personal and family history of obesity, a family history of affective disorders and a family history of substance misuse. Half have a previous history of anorexia nervosa and the aetiology of the two conditions is similar.

ASSOCIATIONS/RISK FACTORS   High prevalence of depression, deliberate self-harm, impulsivity, substance abuse.

EPIDEMIOLOGY   Prevalence amongst adolescent and young adult females is 1–3%. Sex ratio F:M = 10 : 1. Average age of onset is 18 years.

HISTORY   There is a persistent preoccupation with eating and a craving for food. Binge eating of up to 20,000 kcal in one session occurs. This is followed by self-loathing, vomiting and/or laxative abuse and starvation.

EXAMINATION   Weight may be normal. Signs of vomiting: dental erosion, finger calluses, calluses on the dorsum of the hand (Russell's sign), parotid swelling. Menstrual abnormalities occur in 50%. Mood may be low, with self-loathing. There will be a preoccupation with body weight and shape. There is more insight than in anorexia and patients are often keen for help.

INVESTIGATIONS   FBC, U&E, LFT, amylase, lipids, glucose, TFTs, Ca, magnesium, phosphate. ECG due to electrolyte abnormalities.

MANAGEMENT

- Nearly all patients can be managed as outpatients
- Medical stabilisation
- CBT
- Interpersonal psychotherapy
- SSRI antidepressants have an antibulimic effect separate from their antidepressant effect, e.g. fluoxetine

COMPLICATIONS

- Cardiac arrhythmia
- Renal failure
- Mallory–Weiss tears
- Oesophagitis

PROGNOSIS   The majority of patients make a full recovery. CBT is effective for more than half of patients. Poor outcome is associated with depression, personality disturbance, longer duration of symptoms, greater severity of symptoms and substance abuse.

Mood disorders – bipolar affective disorder

DEFINITION Also known as manic depression. Involves recurrent episodes of both depression and mania. The recovery between episodes is usually complete and the frequency and pattern of episodes is variable.

AETIOLOGY Genetic factors have a strong contribution to bipolar affective disorder. Heritability is estimated at 85%. MZ:DZ = 80 : 20%. Risk of bipolar illness in first-degree relatives of those with bipolar is approximately 8%.

ASSOCIATIONS/RISK FACTORS Incidence is higher in higher social classes, urban areas and ethnic minority groups. There is an increased risk of manic episodes in the early postpartum period. Relapse rate is high, especially if the first episode is in adolescence or early adult life. Sleep disruption caused by shift working or long-haul flights may precipitate a manic episode in susceptible individuals.

EPIDEMIOLOGY Lifetime risk 1% and 1-year prevalence 1%. M:F = 1 : 1. First episode usually occurs during early twenties and is more commonly mania than depression.

HISTORY
Hypomania

o Persistent mild elevation of mood (>3 days)
o Increased activity and energy
o Decreased sleep
o Talkative
o Overfamiliarity
o Increased libido

Mania without psychotic symptoms

o Elated mood (or irritability) >1-week duration with complete disruption of work and social life
o Increased energy
o Pressure of speech
o Feelings of high creativity and mental efficiency can lead to grandiose ideas. Expenditure can be excessive and lead to debts
o Sexual disinhibition
o Reduced sleep may lead to physical exhaustion

Mania with psychotic symptoms

o Manic symptoms as above
o Delusions are often mood congruent (grandiose)
o Auditory hallucinations may be present

Depression with or without psychotic symptoms
See Depression section below for diagnosis of depressive episodes.

EXAMINATION
Appearance: Dress inappropriate/bright/outlandish. May be neglect of personal hygiene.
Behaviour: Overfamiliar, even flirtatious, increased psychomotor activity. Distractible, restless.
Speech: Loud, pressure of speech, uninterruptible, flight of ideas, puns and rhymes.
Mood: Elated but can quickly turn to irritability and anger.
Thought: Grandiose or persecutory delusions may be present.
Perception: Auditory hallucinations, often mood congruent.

Cognition: Attention and concentration often impaired.

Insight: Poor.

INVESTIGATIONS   Exclude other causes for a manic episode: substance misuse, space-occupying lesion, hyperthyroidism, corticosteroids, anabolic androgenic steroids. FBC, U + Es, LFTs, Ca, TFTs, glucose, urine drug screen.

MANAGEMENT

Acute manic episode	Prophylaxis
• Most patients will require hospital admission – use of MHA if poor insight.	• Many clinicians think that one episode of mania at an early age is an indication for prophylactic treatment.
• Lithium is a mood stabiliser. It takes 3–7 days to achieve therapeutic effect so antipsychotics are required for rapid control of acute behavioural disturbance.	• Lithium and sodium valproate are mood stabilisers and are the main treatments used to prevent relapse. They help prevent both depression and mania; effective for 80% of sufferers.
• A benzodiazepine may also be used as an adjunct.	• Advise women regarding contraception before starting lithium or sodium valproate.
• Olanzapine can also be used as a mood stabiliser and has the benefit of sedating patients in the acute phase.	• Before lithium treatment is started check renal function and TFT. Lithium has a narrow therapeutic range and therefore levels must be carefully monitored. See section on drug treatments.
• ECT is used if exhaustion is becoming life-threatening.	• Olanzapine is now increasingly being used for prophylaxis and has been shown to be effective.
• Antidepressants can precipitate or aggravate a manic episode, so are stopped.	• Carbamazapine and lamotrigine are also effective and may benefit some non-responders.

See Depression section below for management of depressive episodes.

COMPLICATIONS

- 10% of those with bipolar affective disorder commit suicide.
- Alcohol and substance misuse can complicate the picture.
- Non-compliance with prophylaxis is an important issue. Patients often do not comply due to the side effects or a prolonged period of well-being. Abrupt withdrawal of a mood stabiliser carries a high risk of relapse of mania and/or depression (50% of patients relapse within 5 months if lithium is stopped).
- A minority of patients develop rapid cycling of four or more episodes a year.

PROGNOSIS

- Most relapses are associated with poor compliance.
- The majority of those with bipolar affective disorder are well for most of the time as recovery between episodes is usually complete.
- Unfortunately, even with prolonged prophylaxis, 90% of patients will have at least one recurrence of mania and/or depression within 10 years.
- The median duration of an untreated manic episode lasts 4 months. Depression lasts longer with a median duration of 6 months. Usually with time, manic episodes tend to become less frequent and depressive episodes are more common and last longer.
- Long-term prognosis can be poor as each relapse may be associated with hospitalisation, absence from work/education and strain on relationships.

Mood disorders – bipolar affective disorder (continued)

- Over a lifetime it is estimated that patients with bipolar affective disorder will experience twice as many episodes as those with unipolar depression.
- Predictors of poor outcome:
  - o early onset of illness
  - o poor compliance
  - o persistent depressive symptoms
  - o severe mania
  - o family history of non-response
  - o co-morbid personality disorder
  - o substance misuse
  - o rapid cycling (four episodes a year).

Mood disorders – depression

DEFINITION   Mood disorder characterised by a pervasive lowering of mood accompanied by psychosocial and biological symptoms. A typical depressive episode is described in terms of core symptoms, plus additional features in ICD-10 (see History section below). A depressive episode may be further classified – depending on the severity of the symptoms and the impairment of social functioning – as mild, moderate, severe or severe with psychotic features.

AETIOLOGY   Adoption studies support genetic theories. MZ:DZ = 55 : 25%. Overall risk of mood disorder in first-degree relatives is 20%. Biochemical theories include 5-HT dysfunction. Depressed patients can be viewed as having cognitive distortions (e.g. overgeneralisation, personalisation, minimisation) and having negative views of themselves, the world and the future. Most depressive episodes are preceded by adverse life events.

ASSOCIATIONS/RISK FACTORS

- Chronic illness
- Divorce
- Unemployed
- Lack of confiding relationship
- Low self-esteem
- Poor social support
- Low social class

Co-morbidity with other psychiatric problems, e.g. alcohol misuse, anxiety disorders.

EPIDEMIOLOGY   Lifetime risk: 10–20%. M:F = 1 : 2. Onset any time from childhood to old age but on average in thirties for women and forties for men.

HISTORY   Symptoms are present for at least 2 weeks.
Core

o Low mood
o Loss of interest and enjoyment (anhedonia)
o Fatigue

Additional

o Reduced concentration and attention
o Reduced self-esteem and self-confidence
o Ideas of guilt and worthlessness
o Pessimistic views of the future
o Ideas of acts of self-harm or suicide
o Disturbed sleep
o Diminished appetite

Biological symptoms (four required for diagnosis of somatic syndrome)

o Anhedonia
o Lack of emotional reactivity
o Early morning wakening >2 hours
o Diurnal variation of mood
o Psychomotor retardation or agitation
o Marked loss of appetite
o Weight loss
o Marked loss of libido

Mood disorders – depression (continued)

Mild depression – 2 core symptoms and 2 additional symptoms
Moderate depression – 2 core symptoms and 3 additional symptoms
Severe depression – 3 core symptoms and 4 additional symptoms
Severe depression with psychotic symptoms – delusions, hallucinations or stupor

If severe, the patient may have mood-congruent psychotic symptoms, e.g. hallucinations and delusions. The main themes of these abnormal perceptions are worthlessness, guilt, ill health and poverty, e.g. patients may wrongly believe they have cancer or that they have committed a crime and will be punished. Nihilistic delusions are the belief that something ceases to exist (e.g. the world is about to end) and are particularly associated with severe depressive disorder.

Depressive stupor is an uncommon manifestation of depression characterised by a slowing of movement and poverty of speech so extreme that the patient is motionless and mute.

EXAMINATION
Appearance: Signs of neglect, e.g. weight loss, unkempt appearance.
Behaviour: Poor eye contact, downcast eyes, tearful.
Speech: Slow, non-spontaneous, reduced volume.
Mood: Low. May have suicidal ideation.
Thought: Pessimistic, ideas of guilt and worthlessness. Nihilistic delusions or other delusions.
Perception: Second-person auditory hallucinations, often derogatory.
Cognition: Poor concentration.
Insight: Usually good.

INVESTIGATIONS   Blood tests to exclude medical cause, e.g. TFT, FBC, LFT, U&E, Ca, glucose.

MANAGEMENT

- Risk assessment: risk of suicide, risk to others and self-neglect.
- Minimise adverse life events.
- Primary care if mild, psychiatric referral if severe, hospitalise if suicidal/psychotic.
- Drug treatments: antidepressants (TCA, SSRIs); lithium if refractory.
- Antidepressants should be continued for at least 6 months after symptoms have resolved. They may be taken prophylactically following multiple episodes.
- Antipsychotics to treat any psychotic symptoms in relation to the depressive episode.
- ECT if severe or treatment resistant.
- Psychotherapies: supportive, CBT, IPT.

COMPLICATIONS   Social isolation, unemployment, self-harm/suicide, drug/alcohol abuse.

PROGNOSIS

- Lifetime suicide risk is 15%.
- After an initial depressive episode, 90% recover but almost all will have a recurrence within 10 years.
- 10% have a chronic unremitting course.

Obsessive-compulsive disorder

DEFINITION An anxiety disorder in which the patient suffers from time-consuming obsessions and compulsions that interfere with normal everyday life.

AETIOLOGY

- Genetics – 35% of first-degree relatives also have OCD, MZ:DZ = 50–80 : 25%.
- Serotonin dysfunction.
- Frontal cortex and basal ganglia abnormalities.
- Psychoanalytical models see symptoms as arising from conflicting desires and drives.

ASSOCIATIONS/RISK FACTORS

- Anankastic premorbid personality traits found in 70%.
- Co-morbid depression is present in 30% of OCD patients.
- 15% of patients with schizophrenia have an additional diagnosis of OCD.
- Some patients with OCD also have tics.
- There are high rates of OCD in families with Tourette's syndrome.

EPIDEMIOLOGY Lifetime prevalence 2–3%. M = F. Mean age of onset early twenties.

HISTORY Obsessions and compulsions are present on most days for a period of 2 weeks and are not accounted for by the presence of another mental illness such as schizophrenia. The obsessions and compulsions share the following features:

- Acknowledged as originating in the mind
- Persistent, repetitive and intrusive
- Patient tries to resist them
- Not intrinsically pleasurable
- Cause distress and interfere with functioning

Obsessions may be persistent thoughts, images, doubts or impulses. Common content:

- contamination
- bodily fears
- aggression
- orderliness/symmetry.

Compulsions are stereotyped acts, recognised as excessive, unreasonable or exaggerated. If the patient tries to resist doing them, there is a sense of mounting tension that can be immediately relieved by yielding to the compulsion. Often involve:

- cleaning
- checking
- counting
- hoarding.

EXAMINATION Poor concentration if distracted by unwanted thoughts. May show signs of increasing anxiety if prevented from yielding to compulsions. Patients recognise that the thoughts are their own and excessive.

INVESTIGATIONS FBC, U + Es, LFTs, Ca, TFTs.

MANAGEMENT

- Behavioural therapy (exposure and response prevention and thought stopping) helps up to 90% of patients.
- Clomipramine or SSRIs are efficacious in between 50% and 80% of patients. Often symptoms relapse within weeks of discontinuing treatment.

Obsessive-compulsive disorder (continued)

- If there is a lack of response to SSRIs or clomipramine, an antipsychotic can be added.
- Psychosurgery can be used for severe OCD of at least 2 years' duration with severe life disruption that is unresponsive to other treatments.

COMPLICATIONS   Difficulty with relationships, work and social functioning. It may lead to alcohol and substance misuse.

PROGNOSIS   Worse prognosis if male, early onset, severe symptoms, premorbid obsessional personality disorder, life stresses.

Personality disorders

DEFINITION   Personality disorders are characterised by enduring, deeply ingrained, pervasive and inflexible patterns of inner experience and behaviour, which are maladaptive in the individual's culture and lead to distress or impairment of work or social functioning. The patterns of behaviour deviate from the norm and have their onset in late childhood.

AETIOLOGY   There is some evidence of a genetic contribution to personality disorder.

ASSOCIATIONS/RISK FACTORS   Early adversities that are commonly reported by patients with personality disorder only lead to pathology in a minority of those in the population experiencing similar adversity. This suggests an underlying vulnerability in those who develop personality disorders. Early adversities that are commonly reported are social stressors, childhood abuse and dysfunctional families.

EPIDEMIOLOGY   The symptoms begin in late childhood or adolescence but it is unusual for a diagnosis to be made before adulthood. Five percent of the adult population and 40% of psychiatric inpatients have a personality disorder.

HISTORY   Maladaptions may manifest as:

- cognitions
- affectivity
- control over impulses and gratification of needs
- manner of relating to others
- handling of interpersonal situations
- manner of handling stress.

Personality disorders are divided into three clusters.

Cluster A = Odd/Eccentric

- Paranoid
    - Sensitivity to setbacks
    - Suspiciousness and misinterprets people's intentions
    - Bears grudges
    - Suspicious regarding fidelity of partner
    - Tenacious sense of personal rights
    - Excessive self-importance
    - Conspiratorial view of events
- Schizoid
    - Emotional coldness
    - Few activities provide pleasure
    - Limited capacity to express feelings
    - Indifference to praise or criticism
    - Little interest in sexual experience
    - Preference for solitary activities
    - Preoccupation with fantasy
    - Insensitivity to social norms
    - Uninterested in having close friends

Cluster B = Dramatic/Emotional

- Histrionic
    - Shallow and labile affect
    - Self-dramatisation
    - Suggestibility

Personality disorders (continued)

- o Seeks excitement and wants to be the centre of attention
- o Inappropriate seductiveness
- o Very concerned with physical attractiveness
- Dissocial
  - o Blames others
  - o Callous unconcern for others
  - o Gross and persistent irresponsibility
  - o Unable to maintain enduring relationships
  - o Incapacity to experience guilt
  - o Low threshold for violence
- Emotionally unstable: impulsive type
  - o Act impulsively without thought of consequences
  - o Unstable mood
  - o Inability to control anger
  - o Conflict with others
- Emotionally unstable: borderline type
  - o Some of the features of impulsive type present
  - o Chronic feelings of emptiness
  - o Efforts to avoid abandonment
  - o Intense and unstable relationships
  - o Uncertainty about self-image
  - o Self-harm

Cluster C = Fearful/Anxious

- Anankastic
  - o Preoccupation with detail
  - o Perfectionism interferes with completing tasks
  - o Feelings of excessive doubt
  - o Rigid and stubborn
- Dependent
  - o Allows others to make important decisions
  - o Unwillingness to make reasonable demands on others
  - o Feels helpless when alone
  - o Subordination of own needs to those of others
  - o Fear of being abandoned
- Anxious (avoidant)
  - o Feeling of tension and apprehension
  - o Preoccupation with being criticised
  - o Believe they are socially inept and inferior to others
  - o Restrictions in lifestyle because of the need for security

EXAMINATION MSE will vary depending on the features above.

INVESTIGATIONS

- MRI may be indicated if organic causes of personality change are suspected, e.g. frontal lobe tumour, subdural haematoma.
- Careful and thorough assessment should be conducted – collateral history is essential.
- Psychometric assessments such as the Millon Clinical Multiaxial Inventory may be useful.

MANAGEMENT

- Treatment of co-morbid psychiatric disorders, e.g. depression.

- Psychotherapy (the type of psychotherapy and whether it is individual or in a group will be determined by the type of personality disorder and the individual patient).
- Low-dose antipsychotics are sometimes used.
- Antidepressants may be useful in emotionally unstable personality disorder.
- Carbamazepine may be used for episodic behavioural dyscontrol and aggression.
- Therapeutic communities.

COMPLICATIONS

- Subjective distress.
- Adverse effects on relationships/society.
- Depressive illnesses.
- Alcohol and substance abuse.
- Deliberate self-harm and suicide.
- Violence towards others and other criminal activities.

PROGNOSIS The personality disorders have a high morbidity and mortality. There is a similar standardised mortality ratio for personality disorder and for psychosis. The behaviour of those with personality disorders may improve with increasing age but the cognitive and affective symptoms tend to remain.

Personality type	Prognosis
Paranoid	Poor; many continue to have marital, social and occupational difficulties.
Schizoid	Poor; relationship to schizophrenia is uncertain.
Dissocial	Variable prognosis, may improve with age. Co-morbid problems, e.g. abuse of drugs/alcohol, forensic history, result in worse outcome.
Histrionic	May improve with age. Abuse of alcohol and drugs has a poorer prognosis.
Emotionally unstable	May improve with age. Abuse of substances is associated with a poorer outcome. Increased risk of depressive illness. Increased suicide risk.
Anxious	May develop social phobia. Protected environment has a favourable outcome.
Dependent	Good outcome with treatment. Loss of the person they are dependent on has a poorer prognosis.
Anankastic	May go on to develop OCD, may do well at jobs requiring obsessional behaviour, little improvement with age.

Postnatal mental disorders – postnatal blues

DEFINITION   Also known as the baby blues or maternity blues. It is a common psychological problem typically occurring around the third day post partum. It is not a psychiatric disorder and should not be considered abnormal; however, it is included because it is common and must be distinguished from postnatal depression, which is a psychiatric disorder.

AETIOLOGY   Biological theories suggest hormonal changes after birth: sudden decrease in oestrogen and progesterone.

ASSOCIATIONS/RISK FACTORS

- Women who have previously suffered with premenstrual syndrome
- Primigravidae
- Anxiety and depression during pregnancy
- Fear of labour
- Poor social adjustment
- It is not associated with obstetric factors

EPIDEMIOLOGY   Occurs in between half and two-thirds of mothers.

HISTORY   Symptoms begin within the first 10 days post partum, typically from the third to fifth day. Lability of mood is particularly characteristic, with rapid alterations between euphoria and misery. Women may complain of feeling confused but cognitive function is normal. They are frequently tearful and feel tense and irritable.

EXAMINATION   Tearfulness, irritability, emotional lability.

INVESTIGATIONS   Not appropriate.

MANAGEMENT   Medication is not required. Reassurance, explanation and family support are the key features. Antenatal education that provides warning for women and their partners is helpful.

COMPLICATIONS   May upset early bonding and breastfeeding.

PROGNOSIS   Excellent, resolves spontaneously within a few days.

Postnatal mental disorders – postnatal depression

DEFINITION Also known as puerperal depression. Depression arising in the months following childbirth. It is not qualitatively different from depression occurring at other times.

AETIOLOGY

- Psychosocial factors play a major role, e.g. lack of support.
- Biological theories suggest hormonal changes: sudden drop in oestrogen and progesterone levels.

ASSOCIATIONS/RISK FACTORS

- Past psychiatric history, especially depression.
- Psychological problems during pregnancy.
- Family history of postnatal depression.
- Recent adverse life events.

EPIDEMIOLOGY Affects 10–15% of mothers, usually within the first 3 months of childbirth.

HISTORY May have developed insidiously over several weeks or as an exacerbation of the baby blues. Similar features to general depressive illness. Sleep disturbance, energy changes and low libido are less sensitive indicators as these can occur normally after a birth. Cognitive features are more sensitive indicators and are usually based around motherhood, e.g. feels guilty for not coping as a mother, gains no pleasure from the child, feels angry with the child.

EXAMINATION Depressive features (see Depression). There may be obsessional thoughts (often of causing harm to the baby). Thoughts of harming the baby (infanticide is rare but it must always be considered in women with postnatal depression).

INVESTIGATIONS As for depression.

MANAGEMENT

- Assess risk to mother and child.
- Most cases will be mild and do not require psychiatric intervention and respond to additional support and counselling.
- Moderate depression can usually be managed at home, although if severe, admit to a mother and baby unit (may need to use MHA).
- Multidisciplinary care – liaise with GP and midwife/health visitor.
- Antidepressant medication – see Prescribing in breastfeeding.
- Screening for depression should be incorporated into 6-week postnatal check.

COMPLICATIONS

- Bonding failure
- Rejection/neglect of the baby
- Marital/relationship problems
- Detrimental effect on child's language skills, social and emotional development in the first year of life
- Insecure attachments at 18 months
- Maternal suicide
- Infanticide

PROGNOSIS Untreated, 10% have a course lasting longer than 6 months. 90% of cases last less than 1 month with treatment, 4% are still depressed 1 year later.

Postnatal mental disorders – puerperal psychosis

DEFINITION   A psychotic disorder arising after childbirth.

AETIOLOGY   The strong association with bipolar affective disorder implies a genetic predisposition and there may be a specific familial risk for puerperal episodes in bipolar affective disorder.

ASSOCIATIONS/RISK FACTORS

- Past history of puerperal psychosis
- Existing bipolar affective disorder
- Family history of bipolar affective disorder and puerperal psychosis
- Primigravida

EPIDEMIOLOGY   Arises after 1 in 500–1000 births.

HISTORY   Usually arises within a month of delivery and not uncommonly within the first 2 days. The majority of cases are affective in nature. Typically there are rapid fluctuations in mood and an abrupt onset of disturbed behaviour.

EXAMINATION   Usually marked restlessness and fear. Mixture of manic and depressive symptoms. Delusions and hallucinations may be based around the baby, e.g. paranoid delusions that her baby has been swapped with someone else's and auditory command hallucinations instructing her to kill the baby. There is marked perplexity but no detectable cognitive impairment.

INVESTIGATIONS   To rule out delirium due to infection.

MANAGEMENT

- Risk assessment of mother and child.
- Admit to hospital (if appropriate using MHA), preferably a mother and baby unit. Rarely, can be managed at home with frequent reviews involving CPN.
- Medication as appropriate (antidepressants, mood stabilisers and antipsychotics).
- ECT may be used if medication has failed.
- Supportive psychotherapy may be helpful during recovery to help the woman come to terms with and understand the nature of the illness, and to allow her to eliminate any feelings of guilt or failure.

COMPLICATIONS

- Harm or neglect of the child
- Suicide
- Infanticide

PROGNOSIS   Most cases settle within 6 weeks and are fully recovered within 6 months. However, the recurrence rate is over 50% for subsequent non-puerperal psychosis and 25% for subsequent puerperal psychosis, although this is increased for those with a previous psychiatric history or family history.

Reactions to stressful events – abnormal grief reactions

DEFINITION   'Normal' grief reaction following the death of a spouse/close relative may last for up to 2 years. It is often characterised firstly by shock and disbelief, then sometimes feelings of anger, guilt and self-blame. Later, the person may 'pine' for the relative, feel despair and sadness and have pseudo-hallucinations that the person is talking to them. Finally there is acceptance.

'Abnormal grief' is of delayed onset or prolonged duration. The patient may stay at one stage of the grieving process for a long time (shock, disbelief, denial) so that grief is prolonged.

AETIOLOGY   Unknown.

ASSOCIATIONS/RISK FACTORS   Sudden/unexpected death, problems in the relationship resulting in ambivalence to the bereavement, or being unable to grieve due to 'putting on a brave face' for others (e.g. children).

HISTORY   May have a history of difficult relationship with the deceased (e.g. stormy or over-involved). Symptoms such as shock, disbelief, anger, sadness and despair may be severe. May feel depressed or have suicidal thoughts (especially related to a desire to be with the deceased).

EXAMINATION   They show appearance of self-neglect. Mood may be low and they may be experiencing suicidal ideation.

INVESTIGATIONS   None specifically.

MANAGEMENT   Bereavement counselling, CBT. Monitor suicide risk.

COMPLICATIONS   Depression. Substance misuse. Suicide.

PROGNOSIS   Good, almost all will improve with time.

Reactions to stressful events – acute stress disorders

DEFINITION A transient disorder of significant severity which develops in an individual without a mental disorder in response to a severe stressor.

AETIOLOGY Occurs in response to a broad range of stressors of overwhelming importance, e.g. physical/sexual assault, major road traffic accident, war.

ASSOCIATIONS/RISK FACTORS May represent a maladaptive response to stress. There may be a higher incidence in anxious patients.

HISTORY There must be a clear relationship between the stressor and the symptoms. The onset of symptoms is usually within minutes. Feelings of intense anxiety, accompanied by symptoms of autonomic arousal such as sweating, palpitations and dry mouth. There may also be aggression, hopelessness and overactivity.

EXAMINATION Autonomic arousal – tachycardia, hypertension, sweating. Anxious, restless, may wander aimlessly or be hyperactive. Fearful, disorientated and confused.

INVESTIGATIONS Exclude other neuroses, psychoses or organic disorders producing delirium.

MANAGEMENT Remove the stressor if possible. Reassurance. Short-term anxiolytics (e.g. benzodiazepines) may aid sleep and help relieve symptoms.

COMPLICATIONS May progress to PTSD.

PROGNOSIS If the stressor is transient then the symptoms must resolve after 8 hours. If the exposure to the stressor continues then the symptoms must continue to diminish after 48 hours. If they persist, this suggests the patient is at risk of developing PTSD.

Reactions to stressful events – adjustment disorder

DEFINITION Prolonged severe abnormal response to stress beginning within 1 month of a stressful life event and lasting no longer than 6 months.

AETIOLOGY Maladaptive psychological responses to stressful life events, e.g. divorce, being made redundant.

ASSOCIATIONS/RISK FACTORS May be more likely in patients with poor coping skills.

EPIDEMIOLOGY Any age of onset. It has been estimated that as many as 20% of patients attending a psychiatric outpatient clinic could be diagnosed with an adjustment disorder.

HISTORY Precipitated by a psychosocial stressor. The patient has symptoms of anxiety and depression but not severe enough to diagnose anxiety/depressive disorder. Symptoms of anxiety – irritability, increased arousal, insomnia. Symptoms of depression – tearfulness, low mood. But usually no biological features of depression (i.e. decreased sleep and appetite). Adjustment to a terminal illness may follow a similar course to bereavement – shock and denial, anger, sadness and finally acceptance.

EXAMINATION May have increased autonomic arousal (i.e. increased BP and pulse rate). Fearful, anxious, sweating. There may be preoccupation with the event. Concentration may be poor.

INVESTIGATIONS None specifically.

MANAGEMENT Remove stressor if possible. Supportive psychotherapy, teaching about coping mechanisms and problem-solving techniques.

COMPLICATIONS Short-term disruption of work and social life.

PROGNOSIS Symptoms usually improve rapidly following resolution of the cause.

Reactions to stressful events – post-traumatic stress disorder

DEFINITION An intense, delayed, prolonged reaction to an exceptionally stressful event. The event is likely to cause pervasive distress in almost anyone and usually involves the threat of severe injury or death.

AETIOLOGY Traumatic events, e.g. being the victim of violence or personal attack, rape, observer/survivor of civilian disasters, being involved in combat. Cognitive theories include the following.

- The event challenges currently held beliefs, which results in an inability to cognitively rationalise the event.
- Normal processing of emotionally charged information is overwhelmed so memories persist in an unprocessed form, which can intrude into conscious awareness.
- Negative appraisal of intrusive thoughts maintains experience of symptoms over time.

Between 10% and 25% of those exposed to an exceptionally threatening event will develop PTSD. The subjective meaning of the event to the individual appears to be one of the most important factors in determining whether they develop PTSD.

ASSOCIATIONS/RISK FACTORS Vulnerability factors include:

- childhood trauma
- borderline, paranoid or dependent personality traits
- inadequate support system
- recent stressful life events
- female gender
- low social class and poor education
- past psychiatric history.

Depression, anxiety and alcohol and drug dependence are common co-morbidities.

EPIDEMIOLOGY Occurs at any age. Lifetime prevalence between 1% and 3%. Prevalence in high-risk groups such as Iraq War veterans is approximately 30%. High prevalence in asylum seekers and refugees.

HISTORY Occurs within 6 months of the event. Three main groups of symptoms.

- **Hyperarousal**
  - o Persistent anxiety
  - o Hypervigilance
  - o Poor concentration
  - o Insomnia
  - o Irritability
  - o Exaggerated startle response
- **Intrusions**
  - o Flashbacks
  - o Nightmares
  - o Vivid memories
  - o Frequent thoughts of incident
- **Avoidance**
  - o Avoids reminders
  - o Inability to recall some of the events
  - o Poor interest in everyday life
  - o Emotional detachment
  - o Avoids discussing incident

EXAMINATION   May be signs of neglect related to depression, may look anxious, hyper-vigilance. Poor eye contact, tearful. Slow, non-spontaneous speech. Low mood and suicidal ideation. Concentration may be poor.

INVESTIGATIONS   FBC, U + Es, LFTs, Ca, TFTs.

MANAGEMENT

- Screen for co-morbid psychiatric disorders and conduct risk assessment (suicide/neglect).
- CBT involves identifying and challenging dysfunctional thoughts surrounding the traumatic incident and is often combined with exposure.
- Eye Movement Desensitisation and Reprocessing (EMDR) involves the patient recalling traumatic events while in a state of relaxation resulting from focusing their attention on the therapist's voice and following the therapist's rapid finger movements.
- SSRIs can treat all the core symptoms of PTSD.

COMPLICATIONS   Social withdrawal, suicide, alcohol and drug misuse.

PROGNOSIS   About half make a good recovery within 1 year of onset but the rest may have lifelong symptoms.

Schizophrenia

DEFINITION   A psychotic disorder in the absence of organic disease, alcohol or drug-related dependence/withdrawal. Not secondary to elevation or depression of mood. ICD-10 subgroups of schizophrenia: paranoid; hebephrenic; catatonic; simple; residual.

AETIOLOGY   Multifactorial.

- MZ:DZ = 48 : 4%.
- Candidate genes have been identified.
- Siblings of a patient with schizophrenia have a 10% chance of having schizophrenia.
- If both parents have schizophrenia, their child has nearly a 50% chance of having schizophrenia.
- Hypoxic brain injury at birth has been associated with developing schizophrenia.
- Cannabis use can contribute to the development of schizophrenia.
- Neurochemical theories include abnormalities in glutamatergic neurotransmission which interacts with dopamine pathways.
- Imaging studies show decreased cortical volume, especially of the temporal lobe, and enlargement of the lateral ventricles.

ASSOCIATIONS/RISK FACTORS   Schizophrenic symptoms are more common in those with temporal lobe epilepsy and Huntington's chorea.

EPIDEMIOLOGY   Lifetime risk 1%. Prevalence: 0.5–1%. M:F=1 : 1. Median age of onset: males 28 years, females 32 years.

HISTORY   The onset of symptoms may be preceded by a prodrome where the patient becomes withdrawn, anxious, suspicious and irritable with a reduction in normal functioning.

Symptoms must be present for at least a month.

For a diagnosis to be made according to ICD-10, one of the following signs and symptoms must be present:

- Thought echo, thought insertion, thought withdrawal, thought broadcast
- Delusions of control
- Running commentary or voices discussing the patient between themselves
- Persistent delusions

Or two of the following signs and symptoms.

- Persistent hallucinations in any modality
- Thought disorder
- Catatonic behaviour
- Negative symptoms

EXAMINATION

Positive signs and symptoms	Negative signs and symptoms
Appearance: Normal or inappropriate dress, headgear, etc.	Appearance: Poor self-care/unkempt.
Behaviour: Withdrawn or restless and noisy.	Behaviour: Tardive dyskinesia/poor eye contact/apathy.
Mood: Incongruent affect, guarded.	Mood: Flattened/blunted.
Speech: Reflects underlying thought disorder.	Speech: Poverty of speech.

Positive signs and symptoms	Negative signs and symptoms
Thought: *Formal thought disorder:* derailment, loosening of associations, thought blocking. *Thought alienation:* broadcasting, withdrawal, insertion. *Delusions:* persecutory/reference/control/grandiose.	Thought: May be formal thought disorder, may be persistent delusions.
Perception: Third-person auditory hallucinations, running commentary, hallucinations in other modalities.	Perception: May have persistent auditory hallucinations.
Cognition: Orientation often normal, impaired attention and concentration.	Cognition: Specific cognitive deficits.
Insight: Poor.	Insight: Poor.

Groupings of symptoms that have been previously used.

Schneider's first-rank symptoms

- Auditory hallucinations
  - Third person
  - Running commentary
  - Hearing thoughts spoken aloud
- Passivity phenomena
  - Somatic passivity
  - Actions influenced by external agents
  - Thought withdrawal
  - Thought insertion
  - Thought broadcast
- Delusional perception

Bleuler's 4 As

- Autistic thoughts – inner world of fantasy
- Affective incongruity – e.g. smiling when describing a sad event
- Associations loosened – thought disorder
- Ambivalence – conflicting feelings

INVESTIGATIONS Exclude organic cause. FBC, TFTs, glucose, LFTs, U&E, B_{12} and folate, VDRL. Urine drug screen. If neurological symptoms/signs or if first episode: brain imaging and EEG. Neuropsychological testing.

MANAGEMENT

- Risk assessment: risk of suicide, risk to others, self-neglect.
- Consider need for hospital treatment, possibly under the MHA due to lack of insight.
- Involve family/carers, as they need to be supported and educated about the illness.
- Antipsychotics are the mainstay of treatment. A depot is given if compliance is a problem. Choice of antipsychotic will depend on response and side effects (see Drug treatment chapter).
- Clozapine is used for treatment-resistant schizophrenia (two adequate trials of two different antipsychotics, one of which is an atypical, have failed).
- Augmentation of clozapine can be undertaken with other antipsychotics or mood stabilisers.
- CBT for persisting delusions/hallucinations.
- Behavioural family therapy.

Schizophrenia (continued)

- Social/rehabilitation: day centres (social skills training, vocational training, education, help with benefits and housing, outings and recreation).
- Community care: GP, CMHT, crisis team, assertive outreach team. There has been a shift towards mainly community-based care rather than hospital-based care for those with schizophrenia. Well-organised community follow-up that is integrated with hospital services can increase compliance with medication, reduce the need for hospitalisation and reduce social isolation.

COMPLICATIONS   Personal and social cost: hospitalisation, strain on relationships, dropping out of education, time off work/job loss.

PROGNOSIS

- Variable and difficult to predict for any individual
- 10% chronic course
- 20% one episode only
- 35% several episodes with little functional impairment
- 35% increasing impairment with each of several episodes
- 15% lifetime risk of suicide

Good prognosis	Poor prognosis
Old age of onset	Young age of onset
Female	Male
Married	Unmarried
No family history	Family history
No personality problems	Personality problems
High IQ	Low IQ
Precipitants	No obvious precipitants
Positive symptoms	Negative symptoms
Treatment compliance	Poor treatment compliance
Low expressed emotion	High expressed emotion
Acute onset	Insidious onset
Presence of mood component	No mood component

Schizoaffective disorder

There is considerable overlap between schizophrenia and bipolar disorder. Patients are diagnosed with schizoaffective disorder only if they satisfy the criteria for schizophrenia and mood disorder occurring *during the same episode*, but where psychosis is not secondary to mood disturbance. First-degree relatives of patients with schizoaffective disorder have an increased risk for both mood disorders and schizophrenia. Treat mood symptoms and schizophrenic symptoms, e.g. lithium and antipsychotics may be used in combination. The outcome is generally better than for schizophrenia and worse than for bipolar affective disorder.

Delusional disorder

Delusional ideas without persistent hallucinations and not fitting the criteria for a diagnosis of schizophrenia. The most common delusions are persecutory, grandiose, hypochondriacal and jealous. The age of onset is later than for schizophrenia, usually over 40 years of age. It is more common in those who have hearing impairment. Treatment is with antipsychotics. The prognosis is generally poor.

Somatisation disorder

DEFINITION There is repeated presentation of physical symptoms with persistent requests for medical investigations and no physical basis is found and attempts to discuss possible psychological causes are resisted.

AETIOLOGY Patients tend to have a low threshold for worrying about symptoms and consulting doctors. Often such attitudes are acquired during childhood when illness behaviour/role is learnt through family/cultural influences. Patients are more likely to report parental physical illness and to have had more physical illness themselves during childhood. Ten to 20% of first-degree relatives also suffer from the disorder and the MZ:DZ concordance ratios suggest a genetic influence.

ASSOCIATIONS/RISK FACTORS A high proportion of patients with somatisation disorder will also have a personality disorder. Co-morbidity is also high with anxiety, depression and alcohol abuse.

EPIDEMIOLOGY Lifetime prevalence is approximately 0.1%. More common in women. Onset usually before 30 years old. Onset after the age of 40 may suggest depression.

HISTORY

- Multiple, recurrent and frequently changing physical symptoms, e.g. abdominal pain, headache, fatigue, dizziness, pins and needles.
- Symptoms may affect any system but are most commonly:
  - o gastrointestinal
  - o dermatological
  - o sexual
  - o menstrual.
- No physical explanation is found for the symptoms.
- The symptoms are present for more than 2 years.
- Multiple investigations/treatments by different specialists.
- There is persistent refusal to accept the advice and reassurance of several doctors.
- Social or occupational functioning is impaired as a result of the behaviour.

EXAMINATION All patients require a full physical examination when they first present to exclude physical illness.

INVESTIGATIONS Refusal to accept reassurance leads to multiple investigations for organic aetiology of symptoms.

MANAGEMENT

- Patient should be seen by the same doctor each time.
- Treat any associated anxiety or depression.
- It is important to be clear about negative clinical investigations/findings.
- Do not conduct further investigations.
- Acknowledge psychological distress and offer to help with that.
- Elicit childhood experience of illness.
- Explore the relationship between somatic complaints and possible psychosocial causes.
- Encourage coping strategies and letting go of the inappropriate sick role.
- Involve family who may be reinforcing the behaviour.

COMPLICATIONS New symptoms may appear during times of stress.

PROGNOSIS Chronic and fluctuating. Often resistant to treatment.

Substance misuse – assessment
CAGE
The CAGE questionnaire is a screening tool to identify problem drinking. It is brief and non-confrontational, and so is a very useful bedside test. If two or more of the answers are positive, a full alcohol history must be taken.

C: Have you ever felt you wanted to **c**ut down on your drinking?
A: Has anyone ever **a**nnoyed you by criticising your drinking?
G: Have you ever felt **g**uilty about your drinking?
E: Have you ever had an '**e**ye-opener' (a drink first thing in the morning to avoid the symptoms of withdrawal)?

Full alcohol history
Establish a drinking pattern and quantity consumed

- What is drunk (beer, wine, spirits, etc.)? Remember that patients often underestimate this. It helps to go through a typical day adding up what was drunk and when.
- How much is drunk in units?
- How often do they consume alcohol?
- Where are they drinking (home, pub, etc.)?
- At what time do they have their first drink of the day?
- Do they drink steadily or have periods of binge drinking?

Features of alcohol dependence syndrome
More than three during the previous year for diagnosis of alcohol dependence syndrome (ICD-10).

- Difficulties in controlling alcohol intake. 'Do you ever just have one drink?'
- Primacy of drink. 'Is drinking alcohol important to you? Is it often the first thing that comes to your mind, e.g. when planning a social gathering?'
- Compulsion to drink. 'Do you feel an urge to drink?'
- Tolerance. 'Have you found that alcohol has less effect on you than in the past?'
- Withdrawal. 'Do you ever feel shaky and anxious when you haven't had a drink, especially in the mornings? Do you drink to get rid of these shaky and anxious feelings?'
- Use despite evidence of harm. 'What physical problems have you experienced as a result of drinking alcohol? Have you ever tried to give up/cut down on your drinking? Did you seek help (e.g. AA, counsellors)? What happened?'

Establish impact

- Physical
  - o Liver disease
  - o Peripheral neuropathy
- Mental
  - o Depression
  - o Dementia
- Social
  - o Unemployment
  - o Divorce
  - o Debt
- Legal
  - o Drink driving
  - o Drunk and disorderly

Full drug history
Establish a drug-taking pattern and quantity consumed

- What drugs are used?
- How frequently?
- What amount is used?
- How much is spent on drugs?
- How long have they been using at the current level?
- What route is used? Are they injecting?
- What effect are they seeking?

Features of opioid dependence syndrome
Same features as alcohol dependence syndrome above. Withdrawal features include:

o flu-like symptoms
o yawning
o sweating
o dilated pupils
o piloerection.

Establish impact

- Physical
  o Infections, abscesses
  o HIV, hepatitis B and C
- Mental
  o Psychosis
  o Anxiety
- Social
  o Unemployment
  o Divorce
  o Debt
- Legal
  o Drug offences
  o Theft

Substance misuse – alcohol

DEFINITION Alcohol misuse: consumption of alcohol sufficient to cause physical, psychiatric or social harm. Levels of alcohol consumption:

- Low risk: men <21 units/week; women <14 units/week.
- Hazardous drinking (intake likely to increase the risk of alcohol-related harm): men 22–50 units/week; women 15–35 units/week.
- Harmful drinking (this is synonymous with alcohol misuse). A pattern of drinking associated with the development of alcohol-related harm. Men >50 units/week; women >35 units/week.

AETIOLOGY Multifactorial. No specific cause. See risk factors below.

ASSOCIATIONS/RISK FACTORS Genetic factors, culture, religion, family history, availability and price of alcohol, males.

EPIDEMIOLOGY In the UK, 0.5–1.0% drink harmfully. This number has been increasing over the past decade. Overall, 27% of men and 13% of women drink over the recommended 'low-risk' level of 21 and 14 units/week. M:F= 2:1.

HISTORY See Assessment section above.

EXAMINATION Physical examination for alcoholic stigmata and those of chronic liver disease, e.g. palmar erythema, spider naevi, gynaecomastia, peripheral neuropathy, signs of portal hyper-tension.

MSE will depend on the state of intoxication.

Acute intoxication
Appearance and behaviour: Smell of alcohol, unco-ordinated, may have acute injuries.
Speech: Slurred.
Mood: Labile, may be excessively happy or sad.
Thought: Variable.
Perception: None.
Cognition: Slow, impaired judgement.
Insight: May be poor.

Delirium tremens
Usually starts within 48–72 hours after drinking cessation.
Appearance and behaviour: Agitated, tremor, fearful, may have nausea and seizures.
Speech: Confused.
Mood: Labile, may be anxious.
Thought: Delusions.
Perception: Hallucinations or illusions – usually visual.
Cognition: Confused, poor attention.
Insight: Poor.

INVESTIGATIONS Blood alcohol level, GGT, glucose, LFT, B_{12} and folate, FBC, U&E.

MANAGEMENT

- Detoxification if indicated.
  - o Benzodiazepines to prevent seizures and control withdrawal symptoms.
  - o Rehydration and correction of electrolyte disturbances.
- Vitamin supplements: may need IV supplements (Pabrinex) initially followed by oral vitamin B tablets.
- Motivational interviewing.
- Self-help, e.g. AA.

- Address social issues.
- Disulfiram – blocks alcohol dehydrogenase so leads to an unpleasant reaction on drinking. Works best with supervised administration.
- Acamprosate – reduces conditioned aspects of drinking and prevents craving-induced relapses.
- Naltrexone – opioid antagonist. Reduces reinforcing actions of alcohol, i.e. it reduces the pleasure alcohol gives.
- Treat any co-morbid anxiety and depression.

COMPLICATIONS

- **Mental**
  o Anxiety
  o Depression
  o Alcoholic hallucinosis
  o Morbid jealousy
  o Self-harm
  o Memory loss
  o Dementia
- **Physical**
  o GI upsets (gastritis, ulcers, nausea)
  o Hypertension
  o Cardiac arrhythmias
  o Cardiomyopathy
  o Cirrhosis
  o Hepatitis
  o Jaundice
  o Peripheral neuropathy
  o Delirium tremens is precipitated by withdrawal. Someone in delirium tremens may experience confusion, hallucinations, ataxia, fits, delusions and anxiety. High mortality.
  o Wernicke's encephalopathy – ataxia, nystagmus, ophthalmoplegia and acute confusion. Caused by thiamine deficiency, so responds to administration of thiamine. If untreated, may develop into Korsakoff's psychosis – profound loss of short-term memory.

PROGNOSIS Relapsing and remitting. High suicide risk. Depends on support and premorbid personality.

Substance misuse – illicit drugs

DEFINTION *Acute intoxication* – transient disturbance of behaviour, cognition or perception after taking a substance. *Misuse* – maladaptive and recurrent use of substance leading to significant impairment or distress. *Dependence* – opioid dependence has the same features as alcohol dependence as outlined above.

AETIOLOGY Multifactorial, possible neurobiological mechanism. Pre-existing psychiatric conditions, e.g. personality disorders, may increase the likelihood of substance misuse.

ASSOCIATIONS/RISK FACTORS Peer pressure, deprivation, availability of substances, iatrogenic factors, e.g. prescription of benzodiazepines/analgesics long term.

EPIDEMIOLOGY Difficult to assess as people may not be honest about an illegal activity. In the USA 30% of adults admitted to having tried cannabis, 1.5 % had tried heroin.

HISTORY See Assessment section above.

EXAMINATION Will depend on the substance being used; see table below for physical complications.

INVESTIGATIONS Urine drug screen. HIV and hepatitis screening.

MANAGEMENT Intervention is primarily focused around opioid dependence. However, psychological and social interventions will be of benefit for all types of substance misuse.

- Detoxification from opiates:
  - o Lofexidine
  - o Loperamide
  - o Buscopan
  - o Benzodiazepines
  - o Ibuprofen
  - o Metoclopramide
- Motivational interviewing
- Substitution prescribing: methadone, buprenorphine
- Treat any psychiatric co-morbidity

COMPLICATIONS Physical complications are given in the table below. Substance misuse may worsen/precipitate psychological conditions. Social problems – debts, crime, prison, isolation. Infections and blood-borne viruses may be a consequence of injecting drugs.

PROGNOSIS Depends on the substance of misuse. Also depends on social support and level of motivation.

Physical complications caused by substance misuse

Name	Street names	Class and origin	Effects	Risks
Cannabis	Marijuana, weed, puff, hash, ganja, draw, skunk, shit, blow, pot	Class B. Derived from *Cannabis sativa* plant. Smoked or eaten	Relaxation, heightened senses. Lethargy	Affects concentration and short-term memory. Reduced co-ordination, paranoia, anxiety
Cocaine	Coke, charlie, snow, C, white	Class A. May be snorted or injected	Stimulant. Buzz, alert. Confidence. Lasts roughly 30 minutes	Heart problems, chest pain, convulsions, permanent damage to the inside of the nose. Overdose. Psychosis, post-high depression

Name	Street names	Class and origin	Effects	Risks
Crack	Rock, wash, stone	Class A. Smokeable form of cocaine	High, lasts 10 minutes	Heart problems, addictive. After the high – restless, confused, paranoia, psychosis, depression
Ecstasy (MDMA)	E, fantasy, Rolexes	Class A. Tablets. Often white	Alert, senses more intense. Energy. Lasts 3–6 hours	Nausea, sweating, palpitations. Comedown depression. Liver and kidney problems. There have been 60 deaths in the UK
GHB	Liquid ecstasy, GHB	Colourless liquid in bottles or capsules. Swallowed. No smell but a salty taste. Possession is not illegal, but supply is	Sedative. Can produce feelings of euphoria. Effects last up to a day	Sickness, stiff muscles, fits and even collapse. If incorrectly produced, GHB can badly burn the mouth. Very dangerous when mixed with alcohol or other drugs
Gases, glues, solvents	Lighter gas refills, tins/tubes of glue, paints	Sniffed or inhaled	Dizziness, hallucinations. Lasts 15–45 minutes. Drowsy afterwards	Instant death. Nausea, vomiting, blackouts, heart problems. Long-term abuse can damage brain, liver and kidneys
Heroin (diamorphine)	Smack, brown, horse, gear, H, junk, skag, jack	Class A. Opiate analgesic. Brown/ white powder. Snorted, smoked or injected. Controlled drug	Relaxation, drowsiness. Numbness	Very addictive, tolerance, damage to veins from injecting. Risk of HIV, hepatitis B and/or C from sharing needles
Ketamine	Special K, K, vitamin K	Tablets/powder snorted. Prescription-only medication (PoM)	Hallucinatory experiences for up to 3 hours	Numbness, breathing problems and heart failure in excessive doses
LSD	Acid, tabs, trips	Class A. Tiny squares of paper, often with a picture on one side	Hallucinogenic. 8–12 hours duration. Effects depend on the user's mood	Bad trip – intense anxiety, paranoia, feeling out of control. Accidents. Flashbacks. LSD can complicate other mental health problems, such as anxiety, depression and schizophrenia
Magic mushrooms	'shrooms, mushies	Class A. Main type is liberty cap mushroom. Eaten raw, dried, cooked in food, stewed into tea	Similar to LSD. Relaxation. Lasts about 4 hours	Stomach pains, sickness, diarrhoea. Bad trips. Complicate other mental conditions
Phencyclidine	PCP, angel dust	Usually smoked	Euphoria, peripheral analgesia	Impaired consciousness, psychosis

Substance misuse – illicit drugs (continued)

Name	Street names	Class and origin	Effects	Risks
Poppers (amyl/butyl nitrate)	Poppers, TNT, liquid gold	Clear/straw-coloured liquid in a small bottle or tube. Vapour is inhaled	'Head-rush.' Blood vessel dilation 2–5 minutes	Headache. Dangerous for people with anaemia, glaucoma, breathing or heart problems. Fatal if swallowed
Speed (amphetamines)	Speed, uppers, whizz, billy	Class B. Grey or white powder. Snorted, swallowed, injected or smoked. Controlled drug	Stimulant, increases HR and breathing rate. Energy	Comedown tiredness and depression, sleep concentration and memory all affected short term. Panic and hallucinations. Psychosis
Tranquillisers, e.g. diazepam, temazepam	Moggies (mogadon), valium, downers, benzos	Class C. Penalties. Prescription-only medication (PoM)	Calm, relieve tension and anxiety. Drowsiness and forgetfulness	Accidents. Dangerous if mixed with alcohol. Tolerance and dependence

Neuropsychiatry

Epilepsy

DEFINITION Discrete, recurrent abnormality in electrical activity of the brain resulting in behavioural, motor or sensory changes, or changes in consciousness.

AETIOLOGY Unknown; the aetiology of neuropsychiatric symptoms associated with epilepsy is a combination of biological and psychological factors.

ASSOCIATIONS/RISK FACTORS Family history.

EPIDEMIOLOGY Prevalence of active epilepsy is 1%.

HISTORY Usually presents in three stages.

- *Prodrome*: irritability, tension, restlessness, insomnia; may occur days or hours before a seizure.
- *Ictal (during the seizure)*: symptoms depend on type of epilepsy; aura – only for localised fits. May experience acute perceptual changes, depersonalisation, acute mood changes, rising epigastric feelings.
- *Postictal (after the seizure)*: confusional state. May even experience transient paranoid hallucinations.
- *Psychiatric sequalae*: the following neuropsychiatric symptoms may occur in patients with epilepsy.
  - o Personality changes
  - o Psychosis. *Postictal*: occurs after a seizure. *Interictal*: occurs in between seizures and resembles schizophrenia
  - o Depression
  - o Aggressive behavior

EXAMINATION May have clouded consciousness, simple or complex movements or actions, depending on type of epilepsy.

INVESTIGATIONS Aimed at excluding other causes for seizures, e.g. post-traumatic, cerebrovascular, space-occupying lesions, drug/alcohol withdrawal, hypoglycaemia, hypoxia, encephalitis, syphilis, HIV. Diagnosis is usually on clinical grounds. EEG between episodes may be normal, but may help localise the focus of the seizures. Serum prolactin levels are elevated in the 15–20 minutes after the seizure.

MANAGEMENT

- Antiepileptic medication depending on type of epilepsy. Examples of antiepileptic drugs are sodium valproate and carbamazepine (N.B. these can also be used as mood stabilisers).
- Advise the patient not to drive and ensure that the DVLA are informed (follow DVLA guidance on current medical standards for fitness to drive).
- For management of neuropsychiatric conditions, use psychotropics that do not significantly lower seizure threshold.
  - o Treat depression with antidepressants such as SSRIs.
  - o Treat psychosis with antipsychotics such as haloperidol, sulpiride or trifluoperazine.

COMPLICATIONS Suicide.

PROGNOSIS Mortality higher in patients with epilepsy than healthy controls.

Non-epileptic attack disorder

- Dissociative seizures
- Abnormal illness behaviour
- Difficult to distinguish from epilepsy

Epilepsy (continued)

- Usually have past psychiatric history
- Occasionally, history of childhood sexual abuse
- Injuries, tongue biting and incontinence less common
- Shorter postictal confusion and unconsciousness
- EEG usually normal during the attack
- Serum prolactin is not raised immediately after attack
- Management includes early diagnosis and cognitive-behavioural therapy

Head injury and associated psychiatric sequelae

Head injury in itself is a broad subject with many neurological, social and psychological considerations. This section will focus on the psychiatric sequalae of head injury.

AETIOLOGY Head injury.

ASSOCIATIONS/RISK FACTORS In ascertaining the risk of a head injury victim developing psychiatric symptoms, the following questions should be considered.

- **Premorbid**
  - o What was the patient's ability to tolerate stress before the accident?
  - o Does the patient have any premorbid history of psychiatric disorders?
- **Trauma**
  - o What part of the brain was injured?
  - o How much of the brain was injured?
- **Convalescence**
  - o Are there environmental or internal emotional stressors?
  - o Are there ongoing medicolegal issues such as financial compensation?
  - o Has the patient developed epilepsy?

PSYCHIATRIC MANIFESTATIONS

- *Cognitive impairment*: may be progressive
- *Personality changes*: impulsiveness, irritability
- Post-traumatic stress disorder
- Depression with/without anxiety
- Postconcussion syndrome: headaches, dizziness, visual impairments, difficulty concentrating
- Psychosis

HISTORY AND EXAMINATION Depends on nature of head injury and psychiatric sequalae.

INVESTIGATIONS Neuropsychological assessments, neuroimaging and other investigations, depending on nature of head injury and psychiatric presentations.

MANAGEMENT The management of psychiatric presentation of head injury includes the following.

- *Depression*: antidepressants such as SSRIs and tricyclics
- *Psychosis*: with atypical antipsychotics
- *Irritability/agitation*: carbamezapine, sodium valproate
- *PTSD*: psychological treatments, SSRIs

COMPLICATIONS Epilepsy, suicide.

PROGNOSIS Variable; depends on nature and extent of symptoms.

Huntington's disease

DEFINITION   Genetic illness characterised by choreiform involuntary movements and dementia.

AETIOLOGY   Autosomal dominant. Chromosome 4p- multiple repeats of cytosine/adenine/guanine (CAG) sequence. Too few GABA-ergic and cholinergic neurons in the corpus striatum

ASSOCIATIONS/RISK FACTORS   Family history (or may very occasionally be a new mutation).

EPIDEMIOLOGY   4–7/100,000. M = F. Usual onset 40–50 years (wide variation).

HISTORY   Abnormal involuntary movements. Psychiatric symptoms common and include:

- dementia
- depression
- paranoia and psychosis
- behaviour change and irritability.

EXAMINATION
Appearance and behaviour: Abnormal movements.
Speech: Normal.
Mood: May be low or irritable.
Thoughts: Normal or paranoid ideation.
Perception: Hallucinations in associated psychosis.
Cognition: Impaired in dementia.
Insight: Insight may be good preceding dementia.

INVESTIGATIONS   Genetic tests. Children of an affected parent have a 50% chance of inheriting the condition. Relatives may wish to be tested and require genetic counselling.

MANAGEMENT   Symptomatic treatment.

COMPLICATIONS   Suicide risk for patient and their relatives.

PROGNOSIS

- A neurodegenerative condition.
- More severe with early onset.
- Average duration of illness is 15–20 years.
- The chorea is followed eventually by dementia, seizures and death.
- No treatment can prevent progression.

Motor neurone disease

DEFINITION   Lower and upper motor neurone degeneration without sensory symptoms.

AETIOLOGY   Unknown.

ASSOCIATIONS/RISK FACTORS   Unknown but many factors, including viruses (polio) and genetics (chromosome 21), have been considered.

EPIDEMIOLOGY   Onset age 50–70 years. Affects 7/10,000. M : F = 3 : 2.

HISTORY

- Stumbling, spastic gait, foot-drop
- No sensory symptoms
- Sleep disturbance, fatigue
- Psychiatric manifestations: depression, emotional lability (pseudobulbar palsy)

EXAMINATION

- Upper and lower motor neurone signs on examination: increased spasticity and reflexes, muscle wasting, bilaterally symmetrical
- No sensory impairment
- Mental State Examination:

  Appearance and behaviour: May be fatigued, depressed.
  Speech: Normal, depending on cranial nerves being intact.
  Mood: Emotional lability.
  Thought: Normal.
  Perception: Normal.
  Cognition: Mild cognitive deficits may rarely progress to dementia.
  Insight: Good.

INVESTIGATIONS   MRI, LP to exclude structural/inflammatory causes.

MANAGEMENT

- Treat symptoms, e.g. baclofen for spasticity.
- Treat depression with antidepressants.
- Pain control with narcotics may be needed.

COMPLICATIONS   Frontal lobe dementia (very rare).

PROGNOSIS   Progressive disease. Most die within 5 years of diagnosis.

Multiple sclerosis

DEFINITION Disease characterised by multiple plaques of demyelination and axon loss throughout the central nervous system (predominantly white matter).

AETIOLOGY Unknown.

ASSOCIATIONS/RISK FACTORS Areas of the world with temperate climates.

EPIDEMIOLOGY F > M. 20–40 years peak age of onset. 40/100,000 prevalence.

HISTORY

Physical

- Fatigue
- Spasticity
- Motor weakness
- Numbness
- Bladder spasticity: urinary frequency, urgency, incontinence
- Constipation
- Swallowing disorders
- Visual disturbances
- Ataxia

Psychiatric

- Transient mood changes
- Suicidal ideation
- Depression (may be reactive)
- Euphoria (elevation of mood out of keeping with the patient's physical disability)
- Emotional lability
- Memory impairment and other cognitive deficits
- Psychosis, hysteria and hypomania are rare

EXAMINATION
Appearance and behaviour: May be anxious, irritable.
Speech: Normal.
Mood: Low or may be euphoric.
Thought: Usually normal.
Perception: None.
Cognition: Impaired memory, attention, abstract thinking.
Insight: Good.

INVESTIGATIONS MRI scan may show plaques of demyelination. CSF shows increased protein and oligoclonal IgG bands on electrophoresis.

MANAGEMENT

- Beta interferon: reduces frequency of relapses
- Methylprednisolone
- Baclofen (for muscle spasms)
- Antidepressants (for depression)
- Low dose antipsychotics (for psychosis)

COMPLICATIONS Psychosis (rare), epilepsy.

PROGNOSIS Progressive disease. Prognosis worse if older, male or has many early relapses/ early disability.

Parkinson's disease

DEFINITION   Reduced dopaminergic activity in the striatum causing movement disorders: tremor, rigidity, bradykinesia and difficulty starting and stopping walking.

AETIOLOGY   Degeneration of dopaminergic neurones in the substantia nigra.

ASSOCIATIONS/RISK FACTORS   Mitochondrial mutations resulting in reduced ATP. Pesticides and toxins have also been implicated as possible causes. (Neuroleptics and Wilson's disease may cause a similar Parkinsonian syndrome.)

EPIDEMIOLOGY   Affects 0.5% of the population over 65 years. Age of onset: usually 50–70 years.

HISTORY   Resting tremor, rigidity, slow movement, monotonous speech, shuffling steps (festinant gait).

Psychiatric symptoms are common, including:

- depressive symptoms (reactive or due to neurotransmitter abnormalities) in 70%
- cognitive deficits in 10–20%
- psychoses (due to long-term treatment)-paranoid delusions or visual hallucinations

EXAMINATION
Appearance and behaviour: Masklike face, reduced facial expressions, tremor.
Speech: Slow, monotonous.
Mood: Depression in many.
Thought: Rarely have psychotic symptoms, e.g. paranoid delusions.
Perception: Rarely may have abnormal perceptions (visual hallucinations).
Cognition: 10–20% have cognitive deficits.
Insight: Variable.

INVESTIGATIONS   Clinical diagnosis. Exclude medication as the cause of Parkinsonism.

MANAGEMENT

- A wide range of pharmacological and neurosurgical treatments are now available for Parkinson's disease but are beyond the scope of this book.
- Use atypical antipsychotics for psychosis – these are less likely to induce extrapyramidal side-effects.
- Treat depression with nortriptyline (effective in treating depression).
- Acetylcholine esterase inhibitors (Donepezil, Rivastigmine) – may benefit cognition and hallucinations.

COMPLICATIONS   Depression, suicide, dementia.

PROGNOSIS   Progressive condition.

Syphilis

DEFINITION   Infection with *Treponema pallidum*.

AETIOLOGY   Spirochaete infection.

ASSOCIATIONS/RISK FACTORS   Usually sexually transmitted.

EPIDEMIOLOGY   Prevalence decreased following introduction of penicillin, now increasing again.

HISTORY   Need to know sexual history, any contacts also at risk. Four clinical stages.

- *Primary* – local lesion; infected painless hard ulcer at site of infection (usually an abrasion).
- *Secondary* – 1–2 months later. More generalised lesions and fever, lymphadenopathy, rashes.
- *Tertiary* – rare. 1–5 years after primary infection. Granulomas (gummatous lesions) occur in skin and mucosa.
- *Quaternary* – 8–12 years after primary infection. Affects brain and spinal cord and may lead to meningovascular effects, such as delirium and dementia. May progress to tabes dorsalis and/or general paresis of the insane (GPI).

Tabes dorsalis

- Occurs in approximately 20% of cases of GPI
- Lightning pains, especially in the legs
- Sensory ataxia
- Gait disturbances
- Numbness

General paresis of the insane

- Occurs approximately 20 years after initial infection but this may vary (5–25 years)
- Personality changes and irritability
- Dementia
- Depressive symptoms
- Grandiose delusions/expansive ideas about wealth, power or sexual prowess
- Rarely can lead to full-blown schizophreniform illness

EXAMINATION   Depends on the stage of disease and may include the following:

- Tremor
- Dysarthria
- Increased muscle tone and reflexes
- Inco-ordination
- Argyll Robertson pupil: small, irregular pupil with normal reaction to convergence but no reaction to light. Seen in meningovascular syphilis

INVESTIGATIONS

- Venereal Disease Research Laboratory (VDRL) test
- Treponema-specific antibody, e.g. *Treponema pallidum* haemagglutination assay (TPHA)
- Fluorescent treponemal antibody (FTA) test

MANAGEMENT   Procaine penicillin (daily IM injections). May induce neuropsychiatric improvement even in severe disease.

COMPLICATIONS   Cognitive impairment.

PROGNOSIS   Good when detected and treated early.

Wilson's disease

DEFINITION Hepatolenticular degeneration due to copper deposits in various sites throughout the body.

AETIOLOGY Autosomal recessive, chromosome 13.

ASSOCIATIONS/RISK FACTORS Family history.

EPIDEMIOLOGY Rare. 5–30/1,000,000 prevalence.

HISTORY Copper can be deposited in the:

* *cerebrum* – dementia
* *basal ganglia* – tremor, rigid akinetic syndrome, choreo-athetosis
* *liver* – cirrhosis, jaundice, hepatosplenomegaly
* *eyes* – Kayser–Fleischer rings
* *bones* – osteoporosis, osteoarthritis
* *kidneys* – renal impairment.

Up to 60% of patients with Wilson's disease have psychiatric symptoms.

* Behavioural, personality and/or emotional disturbance
* Depression
* Irritability
* Psychosis
* Cognitive changes and dementia

EXAMINATION MSE will depend on which psychiatric features the patient exhibits.

INVESTIGATIONS Serum copper is low, caeruloplasmin levels low, hypodensities in basal ganglia seen on CT scanning.

MANAGEMENT Mainstay of treatment is reduction of copper levels using dietary copper restriction and/or chelating agents such as D-penicillamine. Treat other symptoms adequately as they present.

COMPLICATIONS Movement disorders, renal impairment, cirrhosis.

PROGNOSIS Better if treated early. All symptoms can improve with treatment. Death is from liver failure, variceal bleeding or infection.

Child and Adolescent Psychiatry

Special considerations for assessment

As young people are embedded within families and schools, the multidisciplinary team is an essential component of assessment and management in child and adolescent psychiatry. In addition to the usual team members in adult psychiatry, teachers and educational psychologists have an important role. Liaison with paediatricians is also often key.

Flexibility is crucial when assessing young people and their families. It is common to assess a young person jointly with a multidisciplinary team colleague. The assessment will usually consist of the following components.

Interviewing the family

o The interview room must be large enough to seat the whole family comfortably.
o Take account of the fact that the child may not have a traditional nuclear family and be clear about the roles and relationships of different family members.
o Construct a genogram (family tree).
o Observe how the family interact with each other and communicate.
o Play material must be available for a wide range of ages.

Interviewing the child alone

o Begin by asking about non-threatening topics such as hobbies and friends.
o Move towards obtaining their perspective of the presenting problem (remember, it is usually their parents who have brought them to the attention of mental health services, not them, and so they may not perceive that there is a problem).
o Try to ask open-ended questions as direct questions often result in denial by the child.

Gathering information from other professionals

o Psychological assessment is valuable and will include assessment of general intelligence, educational attainments, development and personality.
o Obtain information from their school and teacher.
o Liaise with social services and check whether there have been any child protection issues.
o Consult the GP or other doctors who have treated the child.

Attachment and development
Attachment theory

- The attachment theory developed by John Bowlby is an important psychological theory that relates to a child's social development.
- Small babies accept separation from their parents without distress.
- At about 6–7 months of age they start to become attached to a particular individual, known as the attachment figure.
- Attachment refers to the tendency of infants to remain close to certain people (attachment figures) with whom they share strong emotional ties.
- Bowlby considered that infant attachment took place in the context of a warm, intimate and continuous relationship with the caregiver.
- Children may not form adequate attachments due to reasons such as prolonged maternal separation or rejecting parents.

Normal attachment behaviours (6 months to 3 years)

- When attachment figures leave the room, the child will cry, call for them and crawl or toddle after them.
- The child may cling hard when anxious/fearful, tired or in pain.
- Hugging, climbing onto their lap.
- Talking and playing more in their company.
- Uses the attachment figure as a secure base from which to explore.
- They will immediately seek contact with the attachment figure after separation.

Abnormalities of attachment

These categories are derived from Mary Ainsworth's Strange Situation Test which considers the child's behaviour following a period of separation from the attachment figure. Children with abnormal attachment are predisposed to later neurotic disorders and other mental health problems.

Anxious-avoidant

- Child ignores mother.
- Few signs of distress when mother leaves child.
- Can be easily comforted by strangers.

Ambivalent

- Extreme distress on parental departure.
- Seeks contact on parent's return but is angry.
- Resists contact with strangers.

Disorganised

- Chaotic behaviour.
- The child displays unusual behaviour on reunion and may even adopt strange postures for long periods.

Development

Psychiatric disorders can affect normal child development. Developmental milestones and their relationship to Freudian stages are shown in the table below.

Age	Social, emotional and behavioural milestones	Freudian stage
0 to 6 months	Smiling, social responsiveness	Oral
6 months to 1 year	Separation anxiety. Puts food in mouth	Oral
1 to 2 years	Self-help skills, feeding, begins to attain continence, symbolic play with toys, stranger shyness	Anal
3 to 5 years	Attains continence, can dress and undress, can play on their own or alongside others, subsequently learns interactive play	Phallic
Middle childhood: 6 years to puberty	Operational thought – practical and tied to immediate circumstances and specific experiences, increased autonomy and involvement with peer group	Latency
Adolescence	Abstract thought develops – reasoning, concepts, testing hypotheses, relate mostly to peer group	Genital

Freud's theories of child development and identity are very much concerned with the body and with family relations. In early childhood, the identity develops progressively through the phases – oral, anal and phallic.

- Oral – mouth is the focus of stimulation and interaction during feeding
- Anal – anus is the focus of stimulation during toilet training
- Phallic – awareness of self (genitals) and gender role

Attention deficit hyperactivity disorder

DEFINITION   Attention deficit hyperactivity disorder (ADHD) is also known as hyperkinetic disorder. It is a severe form of long-term overactivity associated with inattention and impulsivity arising before the age of 6 years.

AETIOLOGY

- 50% risk in MZ twins.
- There is increased conduct disorder and substance misuse in the parents.
- Functional imaging shows frontal metabolism.
- There is dopamine and noradrenaline dysregulation in the prefrontal cortex.

ASSOCIATIONS/RISK FACTORS   Common co-morbidities are conduct disorder, learning difficulties, antisocial behaviour and depression

EPIDEMIOLOGY   Prevalence 1–2%. M:F = 3 : 1.

HISTORY
Hyperactivity-impulsivity symptoms

o Fidgeting
o Interrupts others
o Jumping the queue
o Talking excessively

Inattention symptoms

o Easily distracted
o Does not listen
o Forgetful

EXAMINATION   Development assessment and full neurological screen.

INVESTIGATIONS   Diagnosed by specialist assessment, including psychometric testing. Collect information from parents and teachers to ensure the symptoms are present in more than one environment. Connor's assessment scale may be useful.

MANAGEMENT

- Information and support for parents and teachers.
- Attend to educational deficits and environmental factors.
- Behavioural modification. Educate parents and teachers about appropriate methods – reward good behaviour and discourage reinforcement of problem behaviour.
- Medication (methylphenidate or atomoxetine) under specialist supervision.

COMPLICATIONS

- Difficulties learning (child does not sit still and learn).
- Risk of accidents (due to impulsivity).
- Low self-esteem and peer rejection (behaviours upset other children).

PROGNOSIS   Usually symptoms reduce by puberty. Severe cases may persist into adulthood. Conduct disorder and other co-morbidities give a poorer prognosis and may persist.

Child abuse

DEFINITION   Child abuse includes neglect, emotional, physical and sexual abuse.

ASSOCIATIONS/RISK FACTORS   Unwanted child, mental/physical handicap, young/single parents with their own history of abuse, adverse socio-economic situation.

HISTORY   The following are signs that may alert you to child abuse and will require a fuller assessment.

Physical abuse

o Injuries without convincing explanation
o Bruises of varying ages
o Delayed presentation of injuries
o Injuries inconsistent with the child's stage of development
o Recurrent injuries

Emotional abuse

o Self-harm
o Indiscriminate friendliness
o Immaturity

Neglect

o Failure to thrive
o Inadequate hygiene
o Poor attachment to the parent
o Speech and language delays

Sexual abuse

o Genital trauma or infection
o Highly sexualised behaviour towards adults or children
o Pregnancy
o Unexplained decline in school work or change in behaviour

EXAMINATION   A full physical examination should be performed by a senior doctor skilled in paediatric examination for child abuse. Careful documentation of any injuries, with photographs taken. Height, weight and head circumference should be measured and plotted on a centile growth chart.

MANAGEMENT   Enlist specialist help whenever child abuse is suspected. Contact paediatricians, child psychiatrists and social services child protection teams. Treat specific injuries. The child may need immediate protection; admission to hospital may be appropriate (this allows investigations and MDT assessment). Child protection conference will decide whether to place the child's name on the Child Protection Register, whether there should be an application to the court to protect the child, and what follow-up is needed.

COMPLICATIONS   Vulnerability to conduct, emotional and developmental disorders, as well as depression and parenting problems in adult life.

PROGNOSIS   Women who were sexually abused are at increased risk of psychiatric disorders in general, and in particular borderline personality disorder. Men who were sexually abused may become abusers and perpetuate the cycle.

Conduct disorder

DEFINITION Disorder of childhood or adolescence (below age of 18) characterised by a repetitive and persistent pattern of antisocial behaviours, which violate the basic rights of others and are out of keeping with age-appropriate social norms.

AETIOLOGY Exact unknown. Theories suggested include the following:

Parental

o Violence
o Failure to set rules
o Alcoholism
o Antisocial PD
o Divorce
o Rejection

Child

o Difficult temperament
o Low IQ
o Neurological impairment

ASSOCIATIONS/RISK FACTORS More common in those from deprived areas and children in the care system. ADHD and substance misuse are common co-morbidities.

EPIDEMIOLOGY Prevalence 4%. M:F = 3 : 1.

HISTORY One episode is not significant enough to make the diagnosis; there must be a 6–12-month history. Problems reported by parents or teachers include:

• frequent bad tempers/irritability
• disobedience
• blaming others for their own mistakes
• violence
• bullying
• problems with the police
• inappropriate sexual behaviour.

EXAMINATION MSE may be difficult as they may not engage in conversation. Their behaviour may be disruptive during the interview.

INVESTIGATIONS Check for educational difficulties. Developmental assessment.

MANAGEMENT

• Psychotherapies: family, problem-solving skills, behavioural therapy and group therapies.
• Address educational needs with remedial teaching.
• Provision of alternative peer group activities.
• Parent skills training.

PROGNOSIS Half will develop antisocial personality disorder. Poor prognosis is predicted by early onset, low IQ, co-morbidity, family criminality, low socio-economic status and poor parenting.

Other psychiatric disorders of childhood and adolescence
Bipolar affective disorder
Prevalence in adolescents is approximately 1%. The presentation may be bizarre, mood incongruent and paranoid. Early-onset bipolar affective disorder has a poor prognosis with half showing long-term functional decline.

Depression
Depression is common in young people (8% of male adolescents and 14% of female adolescents) and the risk of suicide makes detection and treatment a priority. Family history is a significant risk factor. Young children present with apathy, failure to thrive, tantrums, separation anxiety and regressive behaviour. Older children present with somatisation, school refusal and sleep disturbance. Adolescents present with low self-esteem, suicidal acts, behavioural problems and biological symptoms of depression. Psychotherapy should be used initially for mild to moderate depression. SSRIs are the first-line medication but should be used at lower initial doses than in adults.

Obsessive-compulsive disorder
Mild subclinical obsessions and compulsions are common and occur in up to a fifth of children. OCD is only usually recognised when severe, although 50% of all cases have their onset by age 15. Presentation and management are the same as in adults.

Schizophrenia
Schizophrenia can have its onset in adolescence. Earlier onset is associated with low IQ. The majority of cases have premorbid abnormalities including developmental delays, learning difficulties and speech and language problems. Thought disorder and hallucinations are common but delusions are rare. About a third later receive a diagnosis of schizoaffective or bipolar affective disorder. When it occurs in this age group, it is usually a chronic severe illness with a poor prognosis. The management principles are the same as for adults.

School refusal
The child refuses to go to school because of anxiety and in spite of parental pressure. It is common around the age of 5 years and 11 years when the change from junior to secondary school may precipitate it. If the problem is acute, the child should be returned to school as quickly as possible but if the problem is chronic then a graded return to school should be arranged. Truancy differs from school refusal in that it is intentional and likely to be associated with other antisocial behaviour.

Sleep disorders
These are common in children: 20% of children have night-time wakefulness, 3% sleepwalk. Night terrors – the child sits up terrified and screaming but cannot be woken enough to reassure. Associated with tachycardia and tachypnoea, may be associated with stress. Usually occur at age 4–7 years, especially in children with a positive family history.

Tourette's syndrome
Characterised by multiple motor and one or more vocal tics. Mean age of onset is 7 years. Facial tics are often the initial symptom. Vocal tics range from sounds to coprolalia (expletives). It is three times more common in boys. It is commonly associated with OCD and ADHD. Management is with CBT and if tics are disabling, medication, such as haloperidol, can be used.

Old Age Psychiatry

Special considerations for assessment

In the UK, specialist services are available for people over the age of 65 presenting with mental health difficulties. Like any other psychiatric referral, assessment of older people with mental health problems relies on eliciting a complete history and completing a physical examination. However, especially with the elderly, the following considerations should be kept in mind.

1. Assessing people in their own environment to get a more complete picture of their cognition and functioning.
2. Enhancing the patient's sensory (hearing aids, spectacles, etc.) and cognitive (familiar environment, right time of the day, etc.) function to facilitate a more complete assessment.
3. Obtaining a good collateral history from various potential sources including the family, GP, district nurses, social services and formal/informal carers.
4. Recognising the important relationship between physical and mental health, especially in cases with delirium, medication reactions and co-morbid medical conditions.
5. Taking a complete physical and drug history.
6. Evaluating more complex issues such as activities of daily living and quality of life.
7. Taking into account issues of carer stress.
8. Assessing the older person's mental capacity to make decisions.
9. Protecting vulnerable adults from abuse (financial, physical and psychological).

A cognitive assessment is an essential component of a psychiatric assessment of any older person. The minimum screening tools to be used are the MMSE (see Section 1) and brief frontal lobe tests.

- Name as many animals as possible in 1 minute (less than 10 is abnormal).
- Explain a proverb.
- Cognitive estimates (requires abstract reasoning, e.g. how many elephants are there in the UK?).

More detailed cognitive assessment can be undertaken as indicated.

Delirium

DEFINITION   An acute, transient, global organic disorder of CNS function resulting in impaired consciousness and attention, thinking, memory, psychomotor disturbances and sleep–wake cycle.

AETIOLOGY   There are many causes for delirium.

- **Cardiovascular:** congestive heart failure, TIA, stroke.
- **Endocrine:** hypoglycaemia, DKA, thyroid dysfunction, Cushing's syndrome.
- **Metabolic:** hypoxia, electrolyte imbalance, dehydration, renal/liver/respiratory failure.
- **Infection:** systemic (UTI, pneumonia, HIV), local (encephalitis, meningitis, syphilis, cellulitis).
- **Trauma:** subdural haematoma, post concussion.
- **Food/nutrition:** thiamine deficiency.
- **Malignancy:** primary and secondary in the brain.
- **Drugs:** anaesthetic (postoperative), analgesics (opiates), anticholinergics, benzodiaze-pines, corticosteroids, digoxin, diuretics, EtOH.
- **Epilepsy:** status epilepticus, postictal states.

ASSOCIATIONS/RISK FACTORS   Extremes of age (old and young), pre-existing dementia, sensory deprivation, unfamiliar environment.

EPIDEMIOLOGY   10% of all hospital inpatients; 30% of elderly hospital inpatients.

HISTORY

- Often collateral history only. Previous mental state important.
- Rapid onset, fluctuating levels of consciousness.
- Symptoms of the underlying cause (see Aetiology above)
- Hypo/hyperactivity (can fluctuate from one to the other).
- Sleep disturbances (insomnia, reversal of sleep–wake cycle).
- Hypersensitivity to light and sound.
- Perceptual disturbance: misidentification, illusions and hallucinations (visual more common).
- Reduced ability to maintain attention to external stimuli.
- Memory impairment, poor registration and retention of new material.
- Anxiety, fear.

EXAMINATION
MSE
Appearance and behaviour: Aggressive purposeless behaviour or drowsy with reduced levels of activity.
Speech: Incoherent, rambling.
Mood: Labile, anxious, depressed, irritable.
Thought: Disordered.
Perception: Illusions, hallucinations and distortions.
Cognition: Memory impairment, disorientation.
Insight: Very limited.

Physical
Autonomic signs – sweating, tachycardia, dilated pupils.

INVESTIGATIONS

- Thorough physical examination, urine screen for drugs, glucose and infection.
- Blood: FBC, U&E, glucose, LFT, TFT, CRP, blood cultures (if appropriate), ABG.

- EEG: generalised slowing of background activity (can be useful for differentiating from depression).
- Depending on clinical findings, other investigations: CXR, HIV test, MRI/CT, LP.

MANAGEMENT   Treat underlying cause.

Medical management

Aimed at managing agitation to facilitate treatment of underlying cause.

- Treat underlying cause.
- Maintain adequate fluid and electrolyte balance.
- Drugs: avoid benzodiazepines unless absolutely essential (as can add to confusion) or for management of alchohol withdrawal.
- Consider use of the MHA if necessary.

Nursing management

- Aimed at reassurance and reduction of disorientation.
- Quiet and reassuring environment.
- Good lighting.
- Avoid frequent changes of staff.
- Encourage relatives/friends to visit.

PROGNOSIS

- Longer stay in hospital.
- Increased mortality: 20–25% in elderly patients.
- Depends on the rapid diagnosis, treatment and prognosis of the underlying cause.

It is important to distinguish between delirium and dementia, particularly in the elderly. However, dementia is a risk factor for delirium, and the two conditions can co-exist. The table below highlights some of the differences.

Feature	Delirium	Dementia
Onset	Acute/subacute	Chronic/insidious
Course	Fluctuating	Stable, progressive
Attention	Markedly reduced	Normal, reduced
Arousal	Increased/decreased	Usually normal
Delusions	Fleeting	Systematised
Hallucinations	Common	Less common
Psychomotor activity	Usually abnormal	Usually normal
Autonomic features	Abnormal	Normal

Dementia

DEFINITION An organic syndrome characterised by deterioration of intellectual functioning in several cognitive domains without impairment of consciousness and this deterioration has an impact on the individual's daily living, occupational and or social functioning.

AETIOLOGY Most common causes (accounting for more than 90% of all cases of dementia):

- Alzheimer's disease
- Vascular dementia
- Diffuse Lewy body dementia
- Pick's disease
- Normal-pressure hydrocephalus
- Prion disease (CJD).

See Neuropsychiatry section for other causes of reduced cognitive function.

ASSOCIATIONS/RISK FACTORS

Type of dementia	Associated pathological findings	Genetic associations	Other
Alzheimer's disease	Generalised atrophy of the brain. Widening of the sulci and ventricles. Extracellular senile (β-amyloid) plaques and intracellular neurofibrillary tangles. Reduced levels of neurotransmitters, e.g. ACh, NA, 5-HT.	E4 variant of apolipoprotein E gene. ? Autosomal dominant mutations causing early-onset familial dementia. APP. Presenilin 1 & 2.	Age – increasing age is single most important risk factor. Family history. Down's syndrome associated with early-onset dementia. Head injury.
Vascular dementia	Multiple white matter infarcts. Cystic necrosis of infarcted areas, reactive gliosis, patches of demyelinisation of white matter.	Unknown.	Hypertension. Diabetes. Smoking. Male. Old age.
Lewy body dementia	Lewy bodies (eosinophilic intracellular structures) in cortical and subcortical neurons.	Unknown.	Parkinson's disease.

EPIDEMIOLOGY Prevalence of dementia:

- 1% in 65–74 year age group.
- 10% in >75 year age group.
- 25% in >85 year age group.

HISTORY Often from a worried family member who has noticed changes in:

- **memory**, e.g. 'leaves the gas on and loses the door keys'
- **behaviour**, e.g. 'doesn't want to go out and visit friends any more like always used to'
- **personality**, e.g. 'used to be a calm person, but now is very irritable and anxious'
- **mood change**, e.g. 'normally very cheerful but nothing seems to give pleasure any more'.

Differentiating between the dementias – the main features

Type of dementia	Age of onset and time course	Key clinical features
Alzheimer's disease	Onset usually after 65 years. Relentlessly progressive. Early onset, more rapid progression.	Short-term memory loss, difficulty learning/ retaining new information. Dysphasia, dyspraxia. Early impairment of sense of smell, persecutory beliefs are common.
Vascular dementia	Acute onset. Stepwise deterioration.	Memory loss, personality change, signs of vascular disease elsewhere.
Lewy body dementia	Average age of onset is 68 years. Variable rate of progression.	Fluctuating cognitive impairment. Visual hallucinations. Parkinsonian symptoms (bradykinesia more than tremor). Sensitive to antipsychotics. Falls.
Frontotemporal dementia, e.g. Pick's disease	Insidious presenile onset usually between 50–60 years. Slow progression.	Early personality changes. Dementia with prominent frontal lobe involvement: coarsening of social behaviour, disinhibition, speech disturbances, apathy/restlessness. Memory is preserved in the early stages.
Normal-pressure hydrocephalus	Average age of onset after 70 years.	Dementia with prominent frontal lobe dysfunction. Urinary incontinence. Gait disturbance.
CJD	Onset often before 65 years. Rapid progression – death within 2 years.	Affects all higher cerebral functions. Dementia associated with neurological signs: pyramidal, extrapyramidal, cerebellar, aphasia.

EXAMINATION   MSE will depend on the type of dementia. See the table above for distinguishing features. Bedside cognitive tests also add to the understanding of the type and degree of dementia and include the MMSE, Addenbrooke cognitive examination (ACE) and the DemTect.

INVESTIGATIONS   Aimed at identifying aetiology.

- Routine blood tests: FBC, U&E, B_{12} and folate, LFT.
- More specialised blood tests: HIV, syphilis serology.
- Brain imaging (CT or MRI) aids in diagnosis, especially in cases with sudden onset or atypical presentation. Cerebral blood flow imaging tests can also help identify the areas of deficit.
- Neuropsychological testing highlights brain regions affected/severity and can aid in diagnosis, risk assessment and management.
- LP: CSF infection screen and pressure (rarely indicated).
- Specialised tests: genetic tests for familial dementia and EEG for prion disease are carried out in special circumstances.

MANAGEMENT

- Explanation of nature of the illness and broad prognosis to both patient and carers.
- Multidisciplinary approach to diagnosis and assessment of specific needs involving psychologists, occupational therapists, physiotherapists and counsellors in addition to psychiatrists.
- Close working with social services to deliver individualised and person-centred care aimed at maintaining the person's dignity and independence. Care package may include home help, day centres, respite residential stays. Regular reassessment is needed to respond to changing needs.

- Support for carers including assessment of carer needs and information regarding support groups.
- Risk management of issues arising as a result of cognitive impairment:
  - fire safety (cooking and smoking)
  - driving (patients diagnosed with dementia need to tell the DVLA about their diagnosis)
  - wandering or getting lost
  - risk of financial abuse (consider lasting powers of attorney, give information regarding various statutory allowances that might be available for people with dementia such as attendance allowance, council tax benefit, etc.).
- Pharmacological treatments
  - *Acetylcholine esterase inhibitors*: can slow progression in Alzheimer's disease with maximum efficacy in moderate stages.
  - *Antidepressants*: to treat co-morbid depression and agitation (citalopram); are also sometimes used to manage behavioural and psychological symptoms of dementia.
  - *Antipsychotics*: can be used to manage behavioural and psychological symptoms of dementia. They should be used with caution as they increase the risk of cerebrovascular accidents in people with dementia and they should be used in the lowest possible dose for the shortest possible time to target specific symptoms.

COMPLICATIONS

- Difficulty and distress for family – the main carer is often another elderly family member.
- Death often due to pneumonia.
- There is a predisposition to delirium.

PROGNOSIS

- The prognosis depends on the underlying cause.
- Younger age of onset usually means poorer prognosis.
- Alzheimer's disease is usually fatal within 10 years of diagnosis.
- Vascular dementia has a worse prognosis, with sudden stepwise deterioration and risk of sudden death from stroke.

Depression

DEFINITION   Whilst the clinical presentation might vary slightly, the definition of depression in the elderly is the same as that in younger adults (see Section 3). It is a mood disorder characterised by a pervasive lowering of mood accompanied by psychosocial and biological symptoms. A typical depressive episode is described in terms of core symptoms, plus additional features (see History section below). A depressive episode may be further classified – depending on the severity of the symptoms and the impairment of social functioning – as mild, moderate, severe or severe with psychotic features. Symptoms present for at least 2 weeks.

AETIOLOGY   Exact unknown; similar biological (monoamine hypothesis, genetic, endocrine, etc.) and psychosocial (personality trait of neuroticism) vulnerability factors as younger adults.

ASSOCIATIONS/RISK FACTORS

- Physical illnesses
- Females
- Stressful life events
- Past history of depression
- Social isolation

EPIDEMIOLOGY   10–15% in the community, higher in care settings and general hospitals.

HISTORY   The illness is similar to the one described for younger adults in Section 3. However, there are some special considerations in older adults.

- Often presents with hypochondriacal symptoms.
- Agitation and anxiety may be prominent.
- Physical complaints are the patient's main focus.
- Complaints of memory disturbance – 'depressive pseudo-dementia'.
- Lack of appetite and reduced food and fluid intake may put patient at greater risk.

EXAMINATION
Appearance: Signs of neglect, e.g. weight loss, dehydration.
Behaviour: Poor eye contact, agitated and restless.
Speech: Slow, non-spontaneous.
Mood: Low.
Thought: Pessimistic, suicidal, obsessions. Ideas/delusions of a hypochondriacal/nihilistic nature.
Perception: Second/third-person auditory derogatory hallucinations.
Cognition: Poor memory, concentration, disorientation; answers 'don't know' on cognitive testing.
Insight: Usually poor, more focused on physical symptoms.

INVESTIGATIONS   Blood tests to exclude medical cause, e.g. TFT, FBC, LFT, U&E, Ca, glucose.

MANAGEMENT
Risk management

- All self-harm episodes (even seemingly minor ones) should be treated as high risk.
- Dehydration and starvation can put older people at significant risk and should be addressed urgently (ECT might be required).
- Deterioration in physical health due to depression.
- May need to use Mental Health Act if insight poor.

Depression (continued)

Pharmacological treatment

- *Antidepressants*: choice of antidepressant guided by side-effect profile. Treat for longer in initiation, continuation and maintenance phase. If no response with two different classes of antidepressants, augment with lithium or consider ECT.
- *Antipsychotics*: treat any psychotic symptoms with antipsychotics. Review need for antipsychotics in the remission phase as should not be continued indefinitely unless there is a clear need.

Psychological treatment

Cognitive-behavioural therapy.

PROGNOSIS   Broadly, outcome as good as younger adults but increased mortality (due to cardiovascular and other causes). Worse prognosis if slower initial recovery, more severe initial depression, psychotic symptoms or duration of illness more than 2 years.

Very late-onset schizophrenia

DEFINITION   Onset of schizophrenia-like symptoms after the age of 60 years.

AETIOLOGY   No significant increase in first-degree relatives. Increased risk in schizoid and paranoid personality types.

ASSOCIATIONS/RISK FACTORS

- Females
- Sensory deficits, including vision and hearing deficits
- Social isolation

EPIDEMIOLOGY   F>M, 7:1.

HISTORY

- Typically female, living alone, with good premorbid educational and professional adjustment but relationship difficulties.
- First-rank symptoms of schizophrenia are rare.
- Persecutory delusions and 'partition' delusions are common (patient believes that animals, materials or radiation can pass through a barrier such as a brick wall, ceiling or door).
- Hearing voices or noises, either simple in the form of banging or a hum or more complex distinct voices saying derogatory things about the patient.
- Low mood can be reported.

EXAMINATION
Appearance: Usually well kempt.
Behaviour: Occasionally hostile and suspicious.
Speech: Normal rate, rhythm and volume.
Mood: Can be low in mood.
Thought: Delusions of a persecutory nature.
Perception: Simple auditory hallucinations or second-person auditory derogatory hallucinations.
Cognition: Some minor deficits on executive functioning but largely intact.
Insight: Poor insight into symptoms as experiences are very real to the patient.

INVESTIGATIONS   To rule out any physical causes for the delusions.

- Blood: FBC, U&E, LFT, TFT, CRP
- Urine: MSU
- CT/MRI if indicated from neurological examination

MANAGEMENT

- Very important to build trust with the patient by regular and consistent input.
- Rather than challenging delusions, acknowledge distress and offer support.
- Treat with antipsychotics in very low doses (10–20% of adult schizophrenia doses).
- May need treatment with low-dose depot injection, if compliance an issue.
- In very rare conditions, may need Mental Health Act.

PROGNOSIS   Good symptomatic improvement can be achieved if compliance can be ensured.

Psychiatry of Learning Disability

Learning disability

DEFINITION   Learning disability (LD) is an impairment of the CNS originating during the developmental period, which usually presents during early childhood with a below-average intellectual performance and reduced ability to acquire life/adaptive skills resulting in social handicap.

Type	Mild	Moderate	Severe	Profound
IQ	50–69	35–49	20–34	<20
Average age of presentation	School age	3 to 5 years of age	Before 2 years of age	Before 2 years of age
Defining features	Limited in school work, but able to live alone and maintain some form of paid employment later in life	Able to do simple work with support, needs guidance or support in daily living	Requires help with daily tasks and capable of only simple speech	Very disabled in all aspects

AETIOLOGY   The cause of many cases of learning disability, especially mild LD, is unknown but they may be associated with the following.

- Genetic
  - Chromosomal (Down's syndrome)
  - Autosomal dominant (neurofibromatosis, tuberous sclerosis)
  - Autosomal recessive (phenylketonuria)
  - Sex linked (fragile X)
- Structural developmental abnormalities: hydrocephalus
- Secondary to brain damage
  - Antenatal (infection, toxic, hypoxic, maternal disease)
  - Perinatal (birth asphyxia, intracranial bleed)
  - Postnatal (infection, injury, epilepsy, hypothyroidism)

ASSOCIATIONS/RISK FACTORS   Social and educational deprivation. Low parental intellect.

Co-morbid conditions include:

- epilepsy
- autism
- cerebral palsy
- hearing impairments
- visual impairments
- psychiatric disorders
- physical disability.

EPIDEMIOLOGY   The overall prevalence of LD is 2% of the population. Of these, 80% are mild, 12% are moderate, 8% are severe/profound.

HISTORY
Presenting complaints in children

- Delay in usual development (e.g. sitting up, walking, speaking, toilet training).
- Difficulty in managing school work as well as other children.
- Behavioural problems.

Learning disability (continued)

Presenting complaints in adolescents

- Difficulties with peers, leading to social isolation.
- Inappropriate sexual behaviour.
- Difficulty in making the transition to adulthood.

Presenting features in adults

- Difficulties in everyday functioning, require extra support (e.g. cooking and cleaning, filling in forms, handling money).
- Problems with normal social development and establishing an independent life in adulthood (e.g. finding work, marriage and child-rearing).

During assessment

- Collateral history from family/carer is essential.
- Enquire about problems antenatally/perinatally/postnatally.
- Ask about family history of LD.
- Take a thorough childhood history, including developmental milestones.
- Assessment of functioning and life skills.
- Neuropsychological assessment including IQ testing.
- Consider associated problems (epilepsy, neurological and physical disabilities).
- Screen for co-morbid psychiatric problems.

EXAMINATION   In addition to MSE, it is important to conduct a full physical examination, including sight and hearing.

INVESTIGATIONS   FBC, U + Es, LFTs, TFTs, glucose, infection screening and serology. EEG and neuroimaging may be indicated. If genetic disorder suspected, arrange for karyotyping.

MANAGEMENT

- Management is a wholly multidisciplinary approach (e.g. psychiatrist, OT, speech and language therapy, nurse, educational support, social support including finance and housing).
- Treatment of co-morbid medical and psychiatric problems is essential, although unnecessary medication should be avoided (as side effects are common and under-reported).
- Give information to family and carers about support groups.
- Behavioural treatments can be used to teach basic skills and alter maladaptive patterns of behaviour.
- Medication should be used with caution due to limited evidence of efficacy and the increased potential for adverse reactions. Low-dose antipsychotics are sometimes used for aggressive or self-injurious behaviours.

COMPLICATIONS   Patients with learning disability have a higher prevalence of psychiatric symptoms than the general population. There can be difficulty in diagnosing psychiatric conditions due to language difficulties and atypical presentations (e.g. schizophrenia may present with simple repetitive hallucinations and persecutory delusions but few first-rank symptoms; in depression, motor and behavioural changes are more key features than verbal expressions of depressed mood).

PROGNOSIS   Chronic problem but the handicap can be modified by social support.

Autism

DEFINITION   Autism is a pervasive developmental disorder. 70% of those affected have mild to moderate LD (there is normal IQ in Asperger's syndrome). Autism is characterised by a triad of features:

- Language and communication difficulties
- Abnormal social interaction
- Restricted and repetitive behaviour, interests and activities

AETIOLOGY   Unknown. No sound evidence for a causal link between MMR vaccine and autism.

ASSOCIATIONS/RISK FACTORS   Associated with genetic disorders, obstetric complications, infections and neurological disorders.

EPIDEMIOLOGY   Prevalence 5 per 1000 individuals. M:F $= 4 : 1$.

HISTORY

- Onset <36 months. 20% develop autistic features after a period of normal development.
- *Early symptoms*: floppiness, poor eye contact, sluggish feeding.
- *Social impairments*: aloofness, lack of interest in people, unresponsive to social cues, poor eye contact, no capacity to share or understand emotions, failure to develop normal attachments.
- *Language abnormalities*: distorted and delayed speech and language development, echolalia, stilted rate and rhythm of speech, impaired use of gestures and facial expressions.
- *Stereotyped or ritualised behaviour*: hand flapping, rocking, restricted and repetitive behavioural repertoire, insistence on routines, resistance to change, obsessions/compulsions especially in adolescence.
- May have isolated exceptional abilities.

EXAMINATION
Appearance and behaviour: Ritualised, stereotyped behaviour. Poor eye contact, aloof. May attach to unusual items.
Speech: Delayed speech, echolalia, stilted rate and rhythm of speech, impaired use of gestures and facial expression.
Mood: Normal.
Thoughts: Obsessions and compulsions.
Perceptions: No abnormalities.
Cognition: Delayed language development.
Insight: Poor.

INVESTIGATIONS   Full multidisciplinary developmental assessment. Rating scales such as the Autism Diagnostic Interview (ADI–R) and the Autism Diagnostic Observation Schedule (ADOS) may be used.

MANAGEMENT

- Treatment of co-morbid problems, e.g. ADHD, epilepsy.
- Speech therapy to improve language skills.
- Behavioural approach to challenging behaviours.
- Social skills training.
- Education and support of family.
- Educational and vocational interventions.
- Medication as indicated for symptom management.

Autism (continued)

COMPLICATIONS   Social isolation. Inability to live independently in the majority.

PROGNOSIS   Lifelong disorder. Better prognosis with early speech acquisition, higher intelligence and signs of diminishing impairments.

Down's syndrome

DEFINITION   Down's syndrome is due to trisomy of chromosome 21 and is the most common genetic cause of LD. Although Down's syndrome is diagnosed at birth, the LD becomes apparent by the end of the first year of life with delayed milestones.

AETIOLOGY   Full trisomy 21 due to non-disjunction occurs in 95% of cases. Translocations and mosaicism account for the other cases.

ASSOCIATIONS/RISK FACTORS   Risk factors for giving birth to a child with Down's syndrome include the mother being over 40, having a previous child with the syndrome and the mother having Down's syndrome. A third of adults with Down's syndrome have a psychiatric illness.

EPIDEMIOLOGY   Incidence is 5 per 1000 living births in women under 35 years of age. It is 0.5 per 1000 for women under 25 and 35 per 1000 for women over 45.

HISTORY   This should cover the aspects described in the Learning Disability section above. It is important to screen for psychiatric co-morbidity.

EXAMINATION   Classic clinical features.

- Protruding tongue
- Transverse palmar crease
- Up-slanting palpebral fissures
- Short stature
- Brachycephaly
- Eyes close together
- Maxilla reduced more than mandible
- Underdeveloped bridge of nose

INVESTIGATIONS   Diagnosis is made on the basis of the physical appearance at birth and chromosomal karyotyping.

MANAGEMENT   As for any cause of a learning disability (see above). In addition, there will be management of the physical complications of Down's syndrome and any associated psychiatric disorder.

COMPLICATIONS   It is a multisystem disorder and conditions associated with Down's syndrome include the following:

- Congenital cardiac defects
- Congenital duodenal stenosis or atresia
- Squint
- Hearing loss
- Hypothyroidism

PROGNOSIS   Those who survive into their 40s develop Alzheimer's disease.

Genetic disorders
Fragile X
Learning disability is usually the first feature detected in males with fragile X and it varies from mild to severe. Common physical features include macro-orchidism (enlarged testes), elongated face, prominent ears, flat feet and high arched palate.

Phenylketonuria
This is an autosomal recessive condition. It is an important preventable cause of severe LD. It is due to deficiency of phenylalanine hydroxylase (long arm of chromosome 12) and is treated by early restriction of dietary phenylalanine. It is diagnosed after birth with the Guthrie test.

Prader-Willi syndrome
Due to a microdeletion of chromosome 15 and results in mild to moderate LD. Other clinical features include over-eating, sleep disorders, self-injurious behaviour and speech abnormalities.

Tuberous sclerosis
Occurs in 1 in 10,000 births and is autosomal dominant. Most patients have severe LD. They also experience seizures and have hamartomas of the CNS and various skin manifestations, including café-au-lait spots.

Velocardiofacial syndrome
This occurs in 1 in 4000 live births and most patients have a microdeletion in chromosome 22. Over half the patients with the syndrome have LD which is usually mild to moderate. There is also an association with schizophrenia and affective psychoses. There are cardiac abnormalities (usually tetralogy of Fallot) and a characteristic facial appearance: receding jaw, wide-spaced eyes, midface hypoplasia and ear abnormalities.

Forensic Psychiatry

Special considerations for assessment

Forensic psychiatry is concerned with the interface between psychiatry and the law. Forensic psychiatrists are therefore involved in assessing patients involved in the criminal justice system. This requires an understanding of legal terms and criminal proceedings, which are discussed later in this section. Forensic psychiatrists are involved in the assessment and management of mentally disordered offenders and other patients who have been violent or who are considered at high risk of violence.

When considering whether patients may behave violently, it is important to remember the factors that influence offending in the general population. The risk of offending is increased by factors such as having a family history of offending, socio-economic deprivation and pro-criminal attitudes amongst peers. Half of all crime is committed by young males under the age of 21.

A forensic psychiatrist will conduct assessments in a variety of settings, including secure hospitals, prisons, police stations and general psychiatric wards. When assessing a patient in prison, there may not be ready access to information about their medical history. It is important to obtain information from the patient's GP or mental health team and details about their current offence and any previous offences from the prosecution paperwork or prison records. Often a forensic psychiatrist will have to decide whether a mentally disordered offender needs to be transferred from prison and treated in hospital. This will occur under different sections of the Mental Health Act, depending on whether the person is on remand (awaiting trial) or has been sentenced (see Mental health legislation section).

Forensic psychiatrists commonly provide reports for the court offering an expert opinion on matters relating to the mental health of the accused. When assessing somebody for the purposes of a court report, it is important to consider the following issues:

- Do they have a mental disorder?
- What is the relationship between any mental disorder and their offending?
- How might treatment of the disorder influence the risk of future offending?
- Does the patient require detention in hospital?
- How might their current mental state impact on their ability to participate in the court process?

Prior to interviewing the patient, the psychiatrist should obtain comprehensive background information from those requesting the report, including witness statements, record of police interview, record of previous convictions and GP records. The report will contain the usual information from a psychiatric history and mental state examination and will also include:

- details of information sources
- details of the alleged offence from the person and available documents
- opinion on the issues outlined above
- recommendations to the court.

Sometimes the psychiatrist has to attend court to provide oral evidence in addition to submitting their written report. In some circumstances, there may be a recommendation to the court that a patient with a mental disorder should receive a hospital disposal rather than a prison sentence. This means that the patient will be treated in hospital instead of being sent to prison.

Violence and mental disorder

There is a public perception that mentally ill patients commonly behave violently and this idea is perpetuated by adverse media coverage and resulting stigma for patients. Serious violent acts by patients with mental illness are actually rare. Nonetheless, there is an association between some mental disorders and violence and so it is an area of importance to psychiatrists.

Most offending by those with a mental illness is minor. However, having a major mental illness increases the likelihood of acquiring a conviction for a violent offence by about eight times.

Schizophrenia

- There is a modest association between schizophrenia and violence.
- Five percent of the perpetrators of homicide have schizophrenia compared with a prevalence in the general population of closer to 1%.
- Psychotic symptoms alone are not sufficient to make patients act violently which is evidenced by the very small proportion of psychotic patients who commit violent acts.
- The factors associated with violence in those with schizophrenia are those that are associated with violence in the general population, for example:
  o young age
  o male gender
  o substance misuse.
- Delusional jealousy and delusions of love are commonly associated with violent behaviour.
- When psychotic patients are violent, family members are more likely to be the victims than when non-psychotic people behave violently.
- Co-morbid alcohol and drug misuse has been reported as particularly prevalent in psychiatric patients in secure settings. Co-morbid substance misuse in patients with schizophrenia has been shown to increase the risk of violence significantly.
- Patients with schizophrenia are more likely to be victims of violence than perpetrators.

Personality disorders

- Personality disorders have a greater association with offending than any mental illness.
- Various aspects of personality disorders may be related to offending:
  o lack of empathy
  o impulsivity
  o disturbed relationships with others
  o emotional instability
  o poor control of anger.

Risk assessment

Assessment of risk of harm to others is an essential component of all psychiatric assessments along with assessment of the risk of self-harm. However, assessment of risk of violence and management of that risk is the primary concern of forensic psychiatry. As discussed above, there are associations between violence and mental disorders. In those with a mental disorder, the following factors are associated with an increased risk of violence to others:

- Previous violence
- Substance misuse
- Poor compliance with treatment
- Poor response to treatment
- Impulsivity
- Behavioural problems in childhood
- Adverse childhood experiences
- Poor employment record
- Unstable relationships
- Lack of insight into mental illness
- Specific threats
- Active symptoms, possibly particularly:
    o persecutory delusions
    o command hallucinations
    o passivity phenomena

Risk assessment should be multidisciplinary and its basis is a thorough psychiatric history and mental state examination. It is also crucial to obtain as much collateral information as possible in order to produce an accurate and detailed formulation. Useful sources of information will include:

- interviews with family members
- review of previous psychiatric notes
- GP records
- school reports
- record of previous convictions.

Several risk assessment tools have been developed to try to improve the prediction of violence in patients with mental disorder.

Following risk assessment, an appropriate risk management plan should be implemented in order to attempt to reduce the risk of violence.

- Short-term management
    o Consideration of admission to hospital and appropriate level of security
    o Use of mental health legislation (including restriction order if relevant)
    o Use of medication
- Long-term management
    o Treatment of modifiable risk factors, e.g. substance misuse
    o Community support, e.g. housing, follow-up, employment
    o Education of patient and family

Risk of violence to others is a dynamic concept and the risk can change over time, particularly in response to changes in mental state. Therefore, the risk assessment should be reviewed regularly.

Structure of forensic services

Forensic psychiatrists work between two systems.

Criminal justice system	Mental healthcare system
Police stations	Inpatient:
Magistrates' courts	Open wards
Crown courts	Local locked (low-security) wards
Remand prisons	Medium-security hospitals
Sentenced prisons	High-security hospitals
	Outpatient:
	CMHT
	Forensic Community Services

The different types of psychiatric inpatient care

Open wards

These are the admission wards in local psychiatric hospitals. There has been an increase in the levels of disturbance in these wards over the past 20 years, because less severely ill patients are now cared for in the community. There is extreme pressure on beds, and rapid patient turnover.

Psychiatric intensive care units

These have locked doors, higher staffing than in open wards and more of the patients are detained under the MHA. These wards are usually located in general psychiatric hospitals.

Low-security hospitals

These provide longer term treatment and rehabilitation than an intensive care unit but have similar levels of security and staffing.

Medium-security hospitals

These have air-locked entrances, locked internal doors, unbreakable windows, secure garden areas, high nurse–patient ratios, and perimeter security. Patients are likely to be prison transfers or on restricted hospital orders. The average length of stay is 2 years.

High-security hospitals

This type of inpatient care is for those who present a grave and immediate danger to the public. They have perimeter and extensive interior physical security. Average length of stay is 8 years. The three high-security hospitals for England and Wales are:

- Broadmoor, Berkshire
- Rampton, Lincolnshire
- Ashworth, Merseyside.

There is one high-security hospital in Scotland which also accepts patients from Northern Ireland: the State Hospital, Carstairs, in Lanarkshire.

Legal terms and criminal proceedings
Fitness to plead

At the time of trial, the defendant may not be capable of comprehending the trial process and evidence sufficiently to plead and defend themselves. In order to be fit to plead, the defendant must have the capacity to:

- understand the nature of the charge
- understand the difference between guilty and not guilty
- instruct a solicitor
- follow the proceedings in court and understand evidence
- be able to challenge a juror.

Fitness to plead is decided by the judge after hearing psychiatric evidence. If the person is deemed unfit, a second jury is brought in for a 'trial of the facts'. In such circumstances, a range of outcomes is available to the court, from absolute discharge to hospital detention. Being unfit to plead is associated with a severe mental illness or mental impairment.

Insanity defence

'Not guilty by reason of insanity.' This is a retrospective diagnosis of the person's mental state at the time of committing the offence. The McNaghten criteria must be met: '*At the time of committing the act, the party accused was labouring under such a defect of reason, from disease of the mind, as not to know the nature and quality of the act he was doing, or if he did know it, that he did not know that what he was doing was wrong*'. The burden of proof lies with the defence (it is their responsibility to provide evidence that the defendant meets the McNaghten criteria) and it is decided on the balance of probabilities. Usually this defence is used when acutely psychotic patients have committed serious violent offences. There are a range of possible disposal options, from absolute discharge to a restricted hospital order.

In Scotland, the insanity defence is broader than that defined by the McNaghten criteria. The criteria were defined in *Lord Advocate v Kidd*. The case states '*There must have been an alienation of reason in relation to the act committed. There must have been some mental defect by which his reason was overpowered, and he was thereby rendered incapable of exerting his reason to control his conduct and reactions. If his reason was alienated in relation to the act committed he was not responsible for the act even although otherwise he may have been apparently quite rational*'. There is a volitional aspect to the defence that is not present in England. Voluntary intoxication is not a ground for the use of the insanity defence. The range of disposals is the same as in England and Wales.

Diminished responsibility

This reduces the charge of murder to manslaughter. The Homicide Act 1957 states: '*Where a person kills or is party to a killing of another, he shall not be convicted of murder if he was suffering from such an abnormality of mind as substantially impaired his mental responsibility for his acts and omissions in doing or being party to the killing*'. This is used most frequently in cases of psychosis and depression but has been used for personality disorder and premenstrual syndrome. The range of outcomes is from probation to life imprisonment.

Infanticide

This is when '*a woman, by any wilful act or omission, causes the death of her child under the age of 12 months if, at the time of the act or omission, the balance of her mind was disturbed by reason of not having recovered from the effect of giving birth, or of lactation*'. She would be deemed to have committed infanticide. This allows the court to pass any sentence in contrast with the mandatory life sentence associated with murder. It is associated with postnatal depression.

Legal terms and criminal proceedings (continued)
Automatism

An automatism is an act committed during grossly impaired consciousness. It has been defined as *'the state of a person who, though capable of action, is not conscious of what he is doing ... i.e. unconscious involuntary action'*. This is a legal rather than medical definition. There are two types of automatism: sane and insane. It is termed insane if the behaviour is likely to recur and is considered to be a disease of the mind, e.g. sleepwalking and epilepsy. Sentence is left to the discretion of the judge. Sane automatisms are once-only events due to external causes, e.g. concussion and confusional states. The only outcome in sane automatism is acquittal.

Psychotherapy

Special considerations for assessment

Psychotherapies are 'talking treatments'. Symptoms are relieved by way of a professional therapeutic relationship. Although there are many different types of psychotherapy, they all have some common features in their approaches to treatment:

- Trust
- Structure
- Empathy
- Feedback
- Testing solutions
- The therapeutic alliance has been shown to be particularly important for positive outcomes and includes:
  - o the ability of the patient to work purposefully in therapy
  - o an agreement between patient and therapist about goals and objectives
  - o the ability of the patient and therapist to form a relationship
  - o the therapist's ability to provide empathic understanding

In order to assess whether a patient is likely to benefit from psychotherapy, it is useful to consider the following factors:

- Efficacy of psychotherapy as a treatment for their disorder
- Ability to talk about their difficulties openly
- Motivation to engage in psychological work
- Ability to identify psychological factors that relate to their difficulties
- Motivation to change their behaviour
- Previous response to psychotherapy, if relevant

It is usual to see the patient on several occasions in order to develop a thorough formulation and assess their suitability for psychotherapy.

There are many different types of psychotherapy and three of those most commonly used are discussed in more detail below. During the assessment, it will be necessary to consider which type of psychotherapy will be most suitable for the patient concerned. Some forms of psychotherapy can be delivered in group settings and this may be a beneficial option for the patient. Group psychotherapy allows patients to learn from each other and the curative effects of group therapy result from factors such as instillation of hope, imparting of information, catharsis, altruism and imitative behaviour.

Cognitive-behavioural therapy

Cognitive-behavioural therapy (CBT) is structured, time limited and problem and goal orientated. The emphasis is on current problems rather than considering the past. Homework is important and there is a focus on relapse prevention procedures. CBT aims to 'change the way you feel by changing the way you think'. The rationale is that some distressing emotions and behaviours are the result of cognitive errors. These cognitive distortions relate to self, world and future (known as Beck's cognitive triad).

Cognitive methods

- The ABC method involves identifying the **A**ntecedent, the **B**ehaviour and the **C**onsequences. For example, **A** = a panic attack in the supermarket, **B** = avoiding going to the supermarket, **C** = increasing isolation and reinforcement of panic attack.
- Identifying negative automatic thoughts.
  - o *Selective abstraction*: focusing on one minor aspect of the bigger picture.
  - o *All-or-nothing thinking*: thinking of things in absolute terms.
  - o *Magnification/minimisation*: faulty evaluation of relative significance of particular events.
  - o *Catastrophic thinking*: anticipating the worse possible outcome for a situation.
  - o *Overgeneralisation*: if one thing has gone wrong, all others will as well.
  - o *Arbitrary inference*: coming to a conclusion in the absence of any evidence to support it.
- Thoughts diary to recognise connections between cognitions, emotions and behaviour.
- Examine evidence for and against negative automatic thoughts and substitute other more realistic interpretations.

Behavioural methods

- Relaxation techniques.
- Systematic desensitisation involves constructing a hierarchy of anxiety-provoking situations and the patient is exposed to these situations in a graded manner. The exposure can be in their imagination or in real life or a combination of the two, depending on the availability of the phobic object. Patients gradually habituate to the anxiety they experience and the anxiety will eventually be easier to tolerate and subside.
- Flooding involves the patient being exposed to the phobic object without any attempt to reduce anxiety beforehand and they are required to continue exposure until the associated anxiety reduces.
- Activity scheduling (e.g. to combat poor motivation in depression).

Indications

Cognitive-behavioural therapy has been evaluated in randomised controlled trials and has been shown to be effective in the treatment of:

- depression (it is as effective as medication in mild to moderate depressive illness)
- eating disorders
- anxiety disorders
- OCD
- post-traumatic stress disorder
- chronic psychotic symptoms.

In addition, CBT has been shown to reduce the likelihood of subsequent relapse.

Psychodynamic psychotherapy

Psychodynamic theories were developed by Freud, Jung and Klein. The developmental model stresses that early childhood experiences are crucial in shaping the personality. Treatment involves discussing past experiences and how these have shaped the present situation. Unconscious conflicts are explored and the insight gained aims to change patients' maladaptive behaviour. The main goals of psychotherapy are symptom relief and personality modification through exploration of the unconscious. There is much emphasis on the relationship between the therapist and patient. Therapies can be offered on an individual, couple, group and therapeutic residential community basis.

Transference and countertransference

Transference is the patient's attitudes and feelings towards the therapist. It is the projection onto the therapist of assumptions derived from a previous important relationship in the patient's life (usually in childhood). Transference is a very important way for a patient's difficulties to be understood as these relationship problems are re-enacted within therapy. Analysis and interpretation of this transference are the basis of the therapeutic model of psychodynamic psychotherapy.

Countertransference is the therapist's emotional response to the patient. If understood properly, it can allow the therapist to gain valuable insight into the way the patient relates to others.

Defence mechanisms

Defence mechanisms are psychological strategies to protect people from emotional distress. They are utilised unconsciously by everybody at some time to cope with stressful situations. The defence mechanisms are grouped into three categories: mature, neurotic and immature (see below for examples). Those who use mature defences have a better, more stable outcome. An analysis of a patient's use of defence mechanisms can be a useful tool in therapy.

Mature

o Altruism – meeting own needs by helping others
o Humour – seeing the funny side of difficult situations
o Sublimation – modifying unacceptable desires to make them acceptable

Neurotic

o Displacement – transfer of negative feelings to someone/something else
o Reaction formation – opposite reaction to hide true feelings
o Isolation – exclusion of others to protect self
o Repression – thoughts are prevented from being made conscious

Immature

o Splitting – people are either all good or all bad
o Projection – internal issues are attributed to an external cause
o Acting out – unacceptable behaviour in response to conflict, e.g.self-harm
o Passive aggression – anger becomes passive resistance to co-operate

Indications

Dissociative disorders, somatoform disorders, psychosexual disorders, certain personality disorders, chronic dysthymia, recurrent depression.

Relative contraindications

Antisocial personality disorder, acute psychotic disorders, dependence on alcohol or drugs, current depression with high suicide risk.

Supportive psychotherapy

This form of psychotherapy is widely used and has various definitions. The term is commonly used to describe the psychological support given by mental health professionals to patients with chronic and disabling mental illnesses. The objectives of such an approach include optimising the patient's psychological and social functioning, helping them cope with the effects of their illness, increasing self-esteem and self-confidence, education about their illness and the prevention of relapse.

Elements of supportive psychotherapy

Interview

It is now widely recognised that the interview itself can be therapeutic – the act of listening carefully to the patient and allowing them to give a full account of their situation can lead to improvement.

Reassurance

The therapist must be compassionate but also remain objective. It is important not to give false reassurance but fears should be relieved and hope promoted.

Explanation

Discussion of the patient's illness and answering their questions can enhance their ability to cope with their symptoms and their effects on their daily life.

Guidance and suggestion

In this form of psychotherapy it is often appropriate to offer advice or help patients to consider solutions to difficulties they are faced with.

Ventilation

It is important for patients to be able to express their emotions in a safe environment.

Psychopharmacology

Introduction – general points on prescribing

- Always exclude other medical causes that may mimic the underlying disorder.
- Always consider other therapies before prescribing.
- Consider the side effects to ensure the benefits outweigh the risks.
- Choose the appropriate drug based on side-effect profile, e.g. sedating versus non-sedating.
- Consider possibility of withdrawal syndromes or toxicity and risk of overdose.
- When a patient complains of any symptom, look at the drug chart; is it iatrogenic?
- Monitor outcome of the therapy (relapse/improvement).
- Always consider drug interactions when combinations of drugs are prescribed.
- Ensure that the medication you are prescribing does not interact with other medication they may be taking for physical health problems (particularly important for lithium).
- Good communication skills are essential to ensure medication compliance.
- Every patient needs to know:
  - the name of the drug you are prescribing
  - the objective of the treatment – to treat the disease/relieve symptoms
  - how to take and when to take the medicine
  - what to do if they miss a dose
  - how long the drug is likely to be needed
  - how to recognise side effects and any action that should be taken
  - whether there is a need for special monitoring of blood levels of the drug.
- This is a lot for the patient to remember – written leaflets are always helpful.
- This is also a lot for the doctor to remember – always refer to the BNF.
- Refer to the BNF, particularly for special situations, e.g. prescribing for the elderly, for children, in pregnancy.
- For children, the elderly and those with a learning disability you should 'start low and go slow', i.e. use a small dose and increase it very gradually.

Antidepressants – selective serotonin reuptake inhibitors
Examples

- Citalopram
- Fluoxetine
- Paroxetine
- Sertraline

Indications

- Depressive illness (treatment and prophylaxis in recurrent episodes)
- Anxiety disorders (e.g. GAD, panic disorder)
- Bulimia (fluoxetine)
- OCD
- PTSD

Side effects

- Gastrointestinal disturbance (dose related and usually transient)
  - Nausea
  - Vomiting
  - Anorexia
  - Weight loss
  - Diarrhoea
- Sexual
  - Lower libido
  - Delayed orgasm
- Hypersensitivity reactions
- Other
  - Headache
  - Anxiety
  - Sleep disturbance
  - Restlessness

Contraindications

- Mania, use with caution in bipolar disorder

Prescribing notes

- Usually given once a day.
- Used as first line for treatment of depressive illness.
- May take 2 weeks before any effect and 6 weeks for full effect.
- Withdrawal symptoms have been reported (especially with paroxetine).
- Relatively safe in overdose, although some patients have reported increased suicidal ideation initially.

Antidepressants – tricyclic antidepressants
Examples

- Amitriptyline
- Imipramine
- Lofepramine
- Clomipramine

Indications

- Depression
- OCD (clomipramine)
- Neuropathic pain (amitriptyline)
- Nocturnal enuresis in children (imipramine)

Side effects

- Antimuscarinic
  - Dry mouth
  - Blurred vision
  - Constipation
  - Urinary retention
- Drowsiness
- Cardiovascular
  - Postural hypotension
  - Arrhythmias
- Toxicity in overdose
  - Cardiotoxic
  - Respiratory failure
  - Seizures
  - Convulsions
  - Coma

Contraindications

- Recent MI
- Arrhythmias
- Severe liver disease
- Mania – use with caution in bipolar disorder

Prescribing notes

- Given in divided doses or a single dose at bedtime.
- May take 2 weeks before any effect and 6 weeks for full effect.
- May cause drowsiness – advise patients to avoid driving.
- Avoid if high suicide risk in outpatient as can be lethal in overdose (lofepramine is the safest TCA in overdose).

Antidepressants – monoamine oxidase inhibitors
Examples

- Phenelzine
- Moclobemide

Indications

- Refractory/atypical depression

Side effects

- Postural hypotension
- Antimuscarinic
  o Dry mouth
  o Blurred vision
  o Urinary retention
  o Constipation
- Increased appetite and weight gain
- Hepatotoxicity
- Hypertensive crisis – due to interactions between MAOIs and tyramine-containing foods (see prescribing notes). Release of NA causes tachycardia, hypertension and vasoconstriction. May lead to intracerebral or subarachnoid haemorrhage. These hypertensive crises may also be precipitated by:
  o sympathomimetics (cough and decongestant preparations)
  o TCAs
  o amphetamines
  o L-dopa
- Serotonin syndrome – due to interactions between MAOIs and 5-HT enhancing drugs (SSRIs).

NB: Side effects and interactions are less common with moclobemide as it is reversible.

Contraindications

- Mania – use with caution in bipolar disorder
- Hepatic impairment
- Cerebrovascular disease
- Phaeochromocytoma

Prescribing notes

- Patients must carry a card indicating that they are taking MAOIs and must be educated and given written information, especially about dietary requirements.
- Foods to be avoided include:
  o cheese
  o non-fresh fish, meat and poultry
  o broad beans
  o Marmite, Bovril and Oxo
  o alcohol.
- MAOIs should not be prescribed until at least 1 week after cessation of other antidepressants.
- Other antidepressants should not be prescribed until 2 weeks after discontinuing MAOIs.

Antidepressants – others
Examples

- Venlafaxine (serotonin and noradrenaline reuptake inhibitor)
- Mirtazapine (presynaptic α2-anatagonist)
- Trazodone (serotonin antagonist + reuptake inhibitor) – ↑ SE = priapism

Indications

- Depression
- Generalised anxiety disorder (venlafaxine)

Side effects

- Venlafaxine
  o Constipation
  o Nausea
  o Dizziness
  o Sleep disturbance
  o Hypertension
- Mirtazapine
  o Increased appetite and weight gain
  o Oedema
  o Sedation

Contraindications

- Venlafaxine
  o High risk of cardiac arrhythmia
  o Uncontrolled hypertension
  o Pregnancy

Prescribing notes

- Mirtazapine is given at bedtime as it aids sleep.
- Mirtazapine has few antimuscarinic side effects and so can be useful in elderly patients.
- Venlafaxine can be given once daily in a modified-release preparation.
- Venlafaxine should be used as a second-line treatment under specialist supervision.
- Venlafaxine requires monitoring of blood pressure.

Antipsychotics - atypicals
Examples

- Olanzapine
- Risperidone
- Quetiapine
- Aripiprazole
- Amisulpride

Indications

- Schizophrenia
- Other psychotic illnesses
- Mania
- Prophylaxis in bipolar affective disorder (olanzapine)
- Agitation

Side effects

- Weight gain
- Postural hypotension
- Drowsiness
- Extrapyramidal side effects (EPSEs) may still occur but are less common than with typical antipsychotics (see below)
- Diabetes

Contraindications

- Use with caution in those with cardiovascular disease, epilepsy and the elderly.

Prescribing notes

- Monitoring is recommended including:
  - Weight
  - BP
  - ECG
  - Lipids
  - Glucose/HbA1c
  - FBC
  - U + Es
  - LFTs

Antipsychotics - typicals
Examples

- *Phenothiazines* – chlorpromazine, fluphenazine, thioridazine
- *Butyrophenones* – haloperidol, droperidol
- *Thioxanthine* – flupenthixol - b: and name = Depixoi
- *Benzamide* – sulpiride

Indications

- Schizophrenia
- Other psychotic illnesses
- Mania
- Agitation

Side effects
Extrapyramidal side effects (EPSEs)

- Acute dystonia
  - o Presents with grimacing, abnormal movements and facial spasms, especially masseter muscle. May even lead to jaw dislocation, torticollis, limb rigidity and altered behaviour.
  - o Treat with procyclidine 5 mg IM bolus. Symptoms should improve quickly. Then continue with oral procyclidine 8-hourly if necessary.
- Parkinsonism
  - o Tremor
  - o Rigidity
  - o Bradykinesia
  - o Treated with procyclidine or another antimuscarinic drug
- Akathisia (restlessness)
  - o Review medication
  - o Consider propranolol
  - o Difficult to treat
- Tardive dyskinesia (involuntary movements usually of the oral-lingual region)
  - o Consider changing medication
  - o Tends to be irreversible

Neuroleptic malignant syndrome

- A rare but potentially fatal complication of antipsychotic treatments.
- It presents with hyperthermia, fluctuating level of consciousness, muscular rigidity, autonomic dysfunction with pallor, tachycardia, labile BP, sweating and urinary incontinence.
- Increased white cells and creatine phosphokinase.
- Stop antipsychotic and provide cardiovascular and respiratory support (possibly in ITU). Bromocriptine and dantrolene may be used but there is no proven effective treatment.
- Usually lasts for 5–7 days after discontinuation of the antipsychotic.

Prescribing notes

- Monitoring of BP, pulse and ECG is required at regular points throughout treatment.
- To increase compliance, a long-acting depot IM injection can be used (e.g. haloperidol decanoate: one injection every 4 weeks).

Antipsychotics - clozapine
Indication

- Treatment-resistant schizophrenia (psychotic symptoms have failed to respond to adequate trials of two antipsychotics, at least one of which was an atypical)

Side effects

- Agranulocytosis (rare but potentially fatal)
- Constipation (laxatives can be used)
- Tachycardia (can be treated with β-blockers if persists)
- Hypersalivation (can be treated with hyoscine)
- Sedation (give smaller dose in the morning)
- Hypertension (sometimes anithypertensives are needed)
- Weight gain (dietary advice is essential)
- Diabetes (treat accordingly)
- Convulsions (valproate can be given if necessary) (↓ seizure threshold in epileptics)
- Myocarditis

Contraindications

- Severe cardiac disease
- Active liver disease
- Severe renal impairment
- History of bone marrow disorders

Prescribing notes

- Clozapine is very effective and reduces mortality in schizophrenia, largely due to a considerable reduction in suicide rate. However, it can cause considerable side effects. The risk of agranulocytosis is well managed by the mandatory clozapine monitoring systems. These involve the patients having regular full blood counts and the results being checked before the clozapine is dispensed. Blood tests are weekly for the first 18 weeks, then fortnightly for the remainder of the year, then monthly thereafter.
- All side effects are more likely to occur in the early stages of treatment and so careful monitoring is required. Dose should be titrated gradually to minimise difficulties.
- Initiation of clozapine usually occurs while an inpatient but can be done in the community with intensive monitoring.
- BP, pulse and temperature are monitored very closely during titration of dose.
- In addition to intensive titration monitoring and mandatory full blood counts, longer term monitoring requirements include:
  o weight
  o ECG
  o lipids
  o glucose/HbA1c
  o LFTs.
- If the patient misses more than 2 days of their clozapine they will need to be recommenced on their treatment from the beginning with appropriate titration of dose.

Anxiolytics
Examples

- Diazepam, nitrazepam – prolonged action
- Temazepam, lorazepam – shorter action

Indications

- For short-term relief of severe anxiety
- Insomnia (hypnotic effect)
- Alcohol withdrawal
- Status epilepticus (diazepam)
- Premedication before minor surgery

Side effects

- Drowsiness
- Paradoxical agitation and aggression
- Confusion
- Dependence and tolerance with prolonged use so should only be prescribed for the short term
- Withdrawal syndrome after prolonged use:
  o insomnia
  o anxiety
  o loss of appetite and weight
  o tremor
  o sweating
  o perceptual disturbances
  o transfer patient to equivalent daily dose of diazepam and withdraw in gradual steps

Contraindications

- Respiratory depression
- Severe hepatic impairment (benzodiazepines are metabolised in the liver, so accumulation of active metabolites can occur)

Prescribing notes

- Care with alcohol and other minor tranquillisers as they enhance the sedative effects of benzodiazepines.
- Hangover effect can impair the ability to drive or operate machinery.
- Flumazenil is a benzodiazepine antagonist that can be given as an antidote in overdose.
- Administered orally (solutions/tablets), IM, IV, PR in divided daily doses, depending on particular drug used and clinical circumstances.

ADHD medication
Examples

- Methylphenidate
- Dexamphetamine
- Atomoxetine

Indications

- Methylphenidate and atomoxetine– ADHD
- Dexamphetamine – refractory ADHD, narcolepsy
- All should only be prescribed under specialist supervision

Side effects

- Decreased appetite with resultant weight loss and possible growth retardation
- Rebound hyperactivity
- Depression
- Insomnia
- Headache
- GI symptoms (e.g. stomach pain/GI upset)
- Theoretically may worsen epilepsy

Contraindications

- Cardiovascular disease
- Hyperthyroidism
- Predisposition to tics or Tourette's syndrome

Prescribing notes

- Very rarely prescribed in children under 6 years.
- Reserve drug treatment for severe cases that have not responded to other interventions.
- High doses may cause slowing of growth in children.
- Drug may be needed for months to years and careful monitoring of height and weight is essential.
- Need to give 4-hourly doses (morning, lunchtime and possibly evening) as methylphenidate has a short half-life.

Electroconvulsive therapy

- A medical procedure used under controlled conditions to treat some major psychiatric disorders including severe depressive illness, mania, puerperal psychosis and catatonic schizophrenia.
- It is generally used when an illness remains unresponsive to other treatments or when a very rapid response is needed, (e.g. patient not drinking due to depressive stupor).
- The patient is anaesthetised and given a muscle relaxant; seizures are then induced by delivering brief electrical stimuli to the brain via scalp electrodes.
- Patients usually receive a total of 6–12 treatments, given twice weekly.
- The exact mechanism of action is unknown but it is thought to be complex including neurotransmitter release and hormone secretion from the hypothalamus and pituitary.

Special preparations

- The amended Mental Health Act in England and Wales means that ECT can only be prescribed if:
  o the patient understands the treatment and consents
  o the patient does not have capacity to consent and a second opinion approved doctor is consulted and agrees and it does not conflict with an advance directive by the patient.
- Emergency ECT can be given under Section 62 while awaiting a second opinion if:
  o it is immediately necessary to prevent serious suffering
  o it is immediately necessary to prevent the patient presenting a danger to themselves or others.
- Patients must have a full preoperative work-up, including any necessary investigations, e.g. ECG, U&E, CXR and assessment by the anaesthetist.
- Antiepileptics and benzodiazepines should be discontinued before treatment if possible as they increase the seizure threshold.

Practitioners involved

- A nurse who looks after the patient in recovery.
- An anaesthetist who gives the muscle relaxant and anaesthetic.
- A psychiatrist who administers the treatment.

Side effects

- Confusion
- Headache
- Short-term memory impairment

Complications

- Anaesthetic problems (e.g. laryngospasm/tooth damage)
- Status epilepticus
- The risk is the same as that for a general anaesthetic for other minor procedures. (NB: 10% of those with severe depression will commit suicide.)

Contraindications

- Serious anaesthetic risk
- Raised ICP (as ICP rises further during treatment)

Transcranial magnetic stimulation (TMS)

- Based on the principle of delivering focal magnetic fields over specific parts of the cerebral cortex.
- When delivered at high frequency, called rapid-rate TMS or rTMS.

Electroconvulsive therapy (continued)

- Aims to provide more focused stimulation to specific parts of the cerebral cortex to minimise some of the diffuse side effects of ECT.
- Some evidence of benefit in cases of psychotic depression if rTMS applied over the dorsolateral prefrontal cortex.
- Not widely used in the UK at present.

Dementia medication
Examples

- *Acetylcholine esterase inhibitors*: donepezil, galantamine, rivastigmine
- *NMDA receptor antagonists*: memantine

Indications

- Acetylcholine esterase inhibitors:
  - mild to moderate dementia related to Alzheimer's disease
  - mild to moderate dementia related to Parkinson's disease (rivastigmine only)
- Memantine: moderate to severe dementia related to Alzheimer's disease

Side effects

- Acetylcholine esterase inhibitors:
  - *Gastrointestinal*: nausea, vomiting, gastric and duodenal ulcers, GI hemorrhages
  - *Cardiovascular*: dizziness, syncope, bradycardia, AV heart blocks, MI
  - *Psychiatric*: hallucinations, agitation
  - *Others*: rash, muscle cramps
- Memantine:
  - Constipation
  - Hypertension
  - Seizures
  - Dizziness
  - Depression

Contraindications

- Acetylcholine esterase inhibitors:
  - Renal impairment (galantamine)
  - Caution in cardiac disease and those with susceptibility to peptic ulcers
- Memantine:
  - Caution in renal impairment and those with history of seizures

Prescribing notes

- Start with the lowest dose and increase gradually whilst monitoring for side effects.
- With acetylcholine esterase inhibitors, monitor cognition and pulse regularly (at least every 6 months).
- Review appropriateness of acetylcholine esterase inhibitors in severe dementia (MMSE <10).

Hypnotics
Examples

- Zopiclone
- Zolpidem
- Also temazepam and diazepam (see Anxiolytics section above)

Indications

- Short-term treatment of insomnia

Side effects

- Gastrointestinal disturbance
- Headache
- Dependence
- Memory disturbances

Contraindications

- Obstructive sleep apnoea
- Respiratory failure
- Myasthenia gravis
- Pregnancy and breastfeeding
- Caution in history of alcohol or drug abuse
- Caution in hepatic or renal impairment

Prescribing notes

- Before prescribing hypnotics, alternative methods should be attempted, including advice about sleep hygiene.
- Should only be prescribed in the short term (up to 4 weeks).
- Effects of alcohol are enhanced.
- Drowsiness may persist to the next day and impair skilled tasks such as driving.

Medication for alcohol dependence
Examples

- Disulfiram (aversive)
- Acamprosate (anti-craving)

Indications

- Maintenance of abstinence in alcohol dependence

Side effects

- Disulfiram
  - Fatigue
  - Halitosis
  - Reduced libido
  - Rarely psychosis
- Acamprosate
  - GI disturbance
  - Rash

Contraindications

- Disulfiram
  - Cardiac disease
  - Hypertension
  - Previous CVA
  - Psychosis
- Acamprosate
  - Severe hepatic or renal failure

Prescribing notes

- Consuming even a small amount of alcohol while taking disulfiram leads to a build-up of acetaldyhyde, causing an extremely unpleasant reaction, including:
  - facial flushing
  - headache
  - palpitations
  - nausea and vomiting.
- Compliance with disulfiram is increased if it is monitored by a spouse or family member.
- Discontinue acamprosate if the patient returns to regular drinking.

Medication for opioid dependence
Examples

- Methadone
- Buprenorphine (partial opioid agonist)

Indications

- Substitute prescribing for opiates as a means of harm reduction

Side effects

- Methadone
  - Fatal overdose
  - QT prolongation
- Buprenorphine
  - Abdominal pain
  - Fatigue
  - Anxiety

Contraindications

- Caution when prescribing methadone and buprenorphine in those using alcohol and benzodiazepines as this will substantially increase mortality.
- Caution with severe hepatic and renal failure which will reduce the metabolism and elimination of methadone and so increase risk of overdose.
- Methadone is considered safer than buprenorphine in pregnancy and breastfeeding.

Prescribing notes

- Before prescribing, opioid dependence must be confirmed by positive urine results and objective signs of withdrawal (lactorrhoea, rhinorrhoea, agitation, sweating, yawning, dilated pupils).
- The first 2 weeks of methadone treatment are associated with a substantially increased risk of death due to overdose and so careful assessment, titration of doses and monitoring are essential.
- Initial dose is low to reduce risk of overdose and gradually increased depending on withdrawal symptoms.
- Supervised daily consumption of methadone is recommended for the first 3 months.
- In the event of methadone or buprenorphine overdose, naloxone should be administered.
- Commencing buprenorphine may cause precipitated withdrawal and so the first dose should be given when the patient is experiencing withdrawal symptoms to reduce this risk.
- Once patients are stable on buprenorphine or methadone and not using illicit opiates, consideration should be given to gradually reducing the dose with the aim of discontinuing treatment.

Mood stabilisers – carbamazepine
Indications

- Prophylaxis in bipolar affective disorder
- Also used for treatment of epilepsy and trigeminal neuralgia

Side effects

- Erythematous rash may occur in a large number of patients and rarely may be serious
- Gastrointestinal
  - o Diarrhoea
  - o Nausea
  - o Vomiting
  - o Anorexia
- Neurological
  - o Dizziness
  - o Headache
  - o Ataxia
  - o Diplopia
- Haematological
  - o Leucopenia (transient and occurs in 10%)
  - o Thrombocytopenia
  - o Agranulocytosis (1 in 20,000)
  - o Aplastic anaemia (1 in 20,000)
- Biochemical
  - o Hyponatremia

Contraindications

- Atrioventricular conduction abnormalities (unless paced)
- History of bone marrow depression
- Acute porphyria
- Pregnancy and breastfeeding

Prescribing notes

- It may be particularly useful in patients with rapid cycling (four or more episodes in a year).
- Pretreatment investigations are needed:
  - o blood tests – FBC, LFT, U&E
  - o pregnancy test
  - o ECG.
- Regular blood monitoring is required throughout treatment to check FBC.

Mood stabilisers – lithium
Indications

- Prophylaxis in bipolar affective disorder (decreases frequency and severity of manic and depressive episodes)
- Augments antidepressants in treatment of refractory depression
- Mania (use limited by difficulties achieving therapeutic serum levels rapidly)
- Aggressive or self-mutilating behaviours

Side effects

- General
  - Weight gain
  - Fine tremor
  - Muscle weakness
  - Oedema
  - Worsening of acne and psoriasis
- Gastrointestinal
  - Diarrhea
  - Nausea
  - Vomiting
  - Metallic taste
- Renal
  - Nephrogenic diabetes insipidus (polyuria and polydipsia)
  - Long-term use can result in impaired renal function
- Endocrine
  - Hypothyroidism
  - Hyperparathyroidism
- Cardiac
  - T-wave inversion
- Haematological
  - Leucocytosis

Contraindications

- Pregnancy - can cause Ebstein's anomaly (downward displacement of the tricuspid va
- Caution in renal disease and cardiac disease
- Caution in conditions causing sodium imbalance such as Addison's disease

Prescribing notes

- Prescribed only on specialist advice.
- Narrow therapeutic index and possibility of toxic build-up – therefore should only be prescribed after careful consideration of risk:benefit ratio. (Therapeutic range 0.6–1.0 mmol/l. Increased side effects above 1.2 mmol/l. Risk of toxic effects above 1.5 mmol/l.)
- Need pretreatment investigations:
  - medication review (NSAIDs and ACE inhibitors interact)
  - blood tests – FBC, U&E, thyroid screen, pregnancy test
  - ECG.
- Investigations during treatment:
  - lithium plasma levels (every 3 months after dose has stabilised)
  - regular monitoring of FBC, U&E, Ca and thyroid function.
- Advise patients to consume an adequate fluid intake and to avoid diets that may increase or decrease sodium intake.
- Women of child-bearing age should be advised regarding contraception.

- Long-term treatment with lithium reduces the risk of suicide in bipolar affective disorder to the level of the general population.
- There is some evidence that intermittent treatment with lithium may worsen the natural course of bipolar affective disorder and so it should only be commenced if it is intended to continue it for the long term.

Lithium toxicity

Toxic effects occur at levels over 1.5 mmol/l. Antidepressants, anticonvulsants, antipsychotics, diuretics and Ca channel blockers as well as any cause of dehydration can all precipitate toxicity.

Presentation:

- severe nausea
- vomiting
- diarrhoea
- disorientation
- seizures
- drowsiness.

This can lead to coma and death. If lithium toxicity is suspected, the lithium should be stopped and an urgent lithium level obtained and fluids given. Urgent medical attention should be sought as haemodialysis may be needed.

Mood stabilisers – sodium valproate
Indications

- Mania in bipolar affective disorder
- Prophylaxis in bipolar affective disorder
- Refractory depression
- Epilepsy

Side effects

- Nausea
- Vomiting
- Weight gain
- Hair loss
- Rarely hepatic failure
- Pancreatitis
- Pancytopenia

Contraindications

- Hepatic dysfunction
- Porphyria
- Pregnancy and breastfeeding

Prescribing notes

- It may be particularly useful in patients with rapid cycling (four or more episodes in a year).
- Liver function tests should be checked regularly.
- Fewer adverse effects than most anticonvulsants.
- Patients should be given a leaflet about how to recognise haematological/hepatic side effects.
- It is teratogenic and most fetal malformations are neural tube defects. Adequate contraception should be ensured in women of child-bearing age, particularly as manic women may be sexually disinhibited.

Rapid tranquillisation
Examples

- Haloperidol or olanzapine
- Lorazepam

Indications

- Agitation and behavioural disturbance

Side effects

- Acute dystonia
- Sedation
- Extrapyramidal side effects
- Breathing difficulties can occur if held in unsuitable prolonged restraint

Contraindications

- CNS depression

Prescribing notes

- ECG and blood results should be reviewed before prescribing rapid tranquillisation.
- The best response is obtained by using the combination of an antipsychotic and a benzodiazepine.
- Medication should be offered orally first and if this is not accepted, it can be given intramuscularly.
- If patients are elderly, have physical health problems or have never had antipsychotic medication before then the usual doses should be halved.
- Respiration rate, pulse and blood pressure should be monitored every 5 minutes for an hour and then every half hour after administration intramuscularly.
- After rapid tranquillisation there should be a full review of the patient's management to ensure that an appropriate plan is in place.

Appendices

Culture-specific disorders

- A group of psychiatric disorders with diverse characteristics, which were first described in a particular population or culture. They remain closely associated with these populations. However, they do not currently fit into any particular Western classification system of psychiatric disorders.
- It is important to remember that some of the disorders that are categorised in classification systems such as ICD-10 are actually specific to Western culture, e.g. anorexia nervosa, and therefore may be considered culture-bound syndromes by other cultures.
- The table below gives some examples.

Disorder	Associated places	Features
Amok	Indonesia, Malaysia	• Unprovoked episode of destructive behaviour including suicide and homicide, followed by amnesia (the patient has no recollection of the event) and fatigue. • May be precipitated by intense anxiety, hostility or humiliation.
Dhat	India	• Male patients complain of a white discharge in the urine which they attribute to being semen. This is accompanied by features of anxiety. • May be precipitated by excess coitus, urinary disorders, dietary problems.
Koro	South-East Asia, South China, India	• Acute panic or anxiety reaction involving fear of genital retraction and subsequent death. • Precipitants are thought to include interpersonal conflicts, illness, excess coitus.
Latah	Indonesia, Malaysia	• An exaggerated response to fright or trauma characterised by echolalia, echopraxia or trance-like states.
Nervios	Central and South America	• Chronic episode of extreme sorrow or anxiety combined with somatic complaints such as headache, muscle pains, nausea, insomnia. • May be part of a grief reaction or as a reaction to stress, low-self esteem and emotional distress.
Taijin kyofusho	Japan	• Anxiety or phobic disorder. Problems include fear of social contacts, self-consciousness and fear of contracting disease. Somatic symptoms such as headaches and insomnia. • Sufferers are often intelligent and may be perfectionists.

Eponymous syndromes

Asperger's syndrome

A pervasive developmental disorder characterised by abnormalities of social interaction and a restricted, stereotyped, repetitive range of interests/activities. It is part of the autistic spectrum but unlike autism, there is no general retardation in language or cognitive development, and IQ is in the normal range.

Briquet's syndrome

A chronic, severe disorder in which patients present with bodily symptoms that are unexplained by any medical condition. Sufferers are often female and may suffer from anxiety, depression, panic disorder and personality disorders.

Capgras syndrome

A type of delusional misidentification. (See also Frégoli.) Psychotic state characterised by a delusion in which the patient believes a relative or close friend has been replaced by a double.

Cotard's syndrome

Psychotic state characterised by a nihilistic delusion in which the patient believes their body parts do not exist or that they are already dead.

Couvade syndrome

A somatoform-like disorder where expectant fathers experience symptoms resembling those of pregnancy including abdominal swelling, spasms, nausea and vomiting. Anxiety and aching pains are also common.

De Clérambault's syndrome

Also known as erotomania. A psychotic state (classically in women, increasingly seen in men) characterised by unfounded and delusional beliefs that someone else, usually of a higher social or professional status, is in love with them. The patient may make inappropriate advances to the person and become angry when rejected. Some stalkers suffer from this.

Down's syndrome

A genetic disorder – trisomy of chromosome 21. It is the most common cause of learning disabilities.

Ekbom's syndrome

Also known as delusional parasitosis. A psychotic state characterised by delusions in which the patient believes that insects are colonising the body, particularly the eyes and the skin. The patient may present at dermatology clinics or to infectious diseases physicians, requesting deinfestation.

Folie à deux

Also known as induced psychosis. A delusional belief that is shared by two or more people who are closely related emotionally and only one of whom has other psychotic features. The pair are often isolated either in terms of distance or by cultural or language barriers. The psychotic individual tends to be more intelligent and better educated, and often has a dominating influence over the other person.

Frégoli syndrome

A type of delusional misidentification. (See also Capgras.) Psychotic state characterised by a delusion in which the patients believe that strangers have been replaced with familiar people.

Ganser syndrome

A type of dissociative disorder in which the patient gives approximate answers to simple questions, e.g. when asked how many legs a cow has, they may reply seven. Other dissociative symptoms may be present.

Gerstmann syndrome

A name given to a combination of symptoms – agraphia, finger agnosia, acalculia, and confusion of left and right sides – that may occur when the patient has a dominant parietal lobe lesion.

Tourette's syndrome

A disorder in which the patient suffers uncontrollable motor and vocal tics, including blinking, nodding, stuttering, coprolalia, palilalia, echolalia and echopraxia.

Munchausen syndrome

A type of factitious disorder characterised by deliberately feigned symptoms; these may be physical, e.g. chest pain, or psychiatric, e.g. hallucinations. The patient presents many times to hospital clinics and accident and emergency departments. They often give false addresses and have no regular GP. When discovered, they usually appear angry and discharge themselves from hospital against medical advice.

There is a variation of this disorder known as Munchausen syndrome by proxy, in which a mother or carer fakes the illnesses of the child.

Othello syndrome

Also known as delusional jealousy. A psychotic state characterised by a delusion in which the patient (usually male) believes that his spouse is being unfaithful. The patient may go to great lengths to try to produce evidence of the infidelity and is at risk of being violent.

Wernicke–Korsakoff syndrome

These are two different phenomena that can occur together and result from thiamine deficiency; Korsakoff's syndrome may follow Wernicke's encephalopathy. Those affected often suffer from alcoholism.

Korsakoff's syndrome is a reduced ability to acquire new memories (i.e. a loss of short-term memory). The patient confabulates to fill in the gaps. Wernicke's encephalopathy is a disorder of acute onset (hours to days) resulting in global confusion (apathy, disorientation and disturbed memory), eye disturbance (nystagmus and ophthalmoplegia) and ataxia.

Physical disorders – psychological consequences

- **Systemic lupus erythematosus** – psychiatric manifestations can be due to autoimmune reaction to the neurons or the medications used for treatment. Can lead to depression, psychosis, delirium
- **Hyperthyroidism/hypothyroidism** – mania or anxiety/depression.
- **Addison's disease** – reduced cortisol leading to depression, lethargy
- **Cushing's disease** – increased cortisol leading to depression, psychosis
- **Hyperparathyroidism** – increased parathyroid harmone and increased calcium. Can cause cognitive impairment, depression, delirium, psychosis
- **Phaeochromocytoma** – catecholamine-secreting tumour, usually in adrenal medulla. Can lead to anxiety, flushing, palpitations, mimics anxiety disorders
- **Renal failure** – decreased renal function with increase in urea and creatinine levels. *Acute*: delirium. *Chronic*: depression, delirium, dementia
- **B$_{12}$ deficiency** – dementia

Medication – psychological consequences

Some of the common psychological manifestations of medications used for treating physical health disorders are outlined below but the BNF should always be consulted for a full list of up-to-date complications of any medication.

- **ACE inhibitors** depression, mania, psychosis, delirium
- **Amiodarone** sleep disturbance, decreased libido
- **Amphetamines** psychosis
- **β-blockers** fatigue, depression, confusion, psychosis (rarely)
- **Benzodiazepines** delirium, withdrawals, agitation
- **Bendroflumethiazide** anxiety
- **Carbamazepine** depression, cognitive impairment
- **Cimetidine** depression, psychosis
- **Digoxin** psychosis, depression
- **Dopamine agonists** hallucinations, delirium
- **Gabapentin** fatigue
- **Indometacin** depression
- **Ketoconazole** decreased libido, depression
- **L-dopa** visual hallucinations, depression, sleep disorders, delirium
- **Penicillin** confusion, hallucinations
- **Phenobarbital** agitation, depression
- **Phenytoin** agitation, delirium
- **Quinine** delirium
- **Spironolactone** fatigue
- **Steroids** depression, psychosis, mania
- **Topiramate** psychosis
- **Vincristine/vinblastine** depression

Glossary

Abnormal perceptions: abnormalities in the way information from the outside world is sensed and processed, i.e. hallucinations, illusions.

Acute intoxication: changes in physiological and psychological responses due to the administration of a psychoactive substance.

Affect: the behaviour a person exhibits, which reflects the current mood/emotions.

Agitation: feelings of tension combined with excessive physical activity.

Agnosia: patient cannot interpret sensations properly although there is nothing wrong with the sensory organs.

Agranulocytosis: acute deficiency of neutrophils which is a rare side effect of clozapine.

Ambivalence: simultaneous opposing impulses towards something.

Amnesia: inability to recall past experiences/events.

Anhedonia: no longer finding pleasure in previously enjoyable activities.

Attention: the ability to focus on a specific activity.

Blunted affect: reduced expression of emotion.

BMI (Body Mass Index): calculated as weight (kg)/height (m)^2. It is a measure of body weight in comparison to the general population. Normal BMI is in the range 20–25.

Choreiform movements: jerky involuntary movements, particularly affecting the head, face or limbs. They are characteristic of Huntington's disease.

Circumstantiality: a form of thought disorder characterised by speech in which the provision of unnecessary trivial details means that the point of the conversation is reached very slowly.

Clouding of consciousness: the patient is drowsy and does not respond completely to stimuli. There is disturbance of attention, concentration, memory, orientation and thinking.

Cognition: mental processes by which knowledge is acquired and acted on. Includes reasoning, creativity and problem solving.

Compulsion: repetitive stereotyped act performed, despite knowing it is senseless, in order to reduce anxiety, and in response to obsessional thoughts.

Concentration: the ability to maintain attention.

Concrete thinking: lack of abstract thought. Normal in children. Occurs in adults with schizophrenia or organic brain disease, e.g. 'People in glass houses shouldn't throw stones – because they would break the windows'.

Confabulation: gaps in memory are unconsciously filled with false memories/explanations.

Coprolalia: the repetitive speaking of obscene words.

Countertransference: the therapist's emotions and attitudes to the patient.

Defence mechanism: mental mechanisms that protect the consciousness from the affects, ideas and desires of the unconscious.

Déjà vu: illusion of familiarity of a situation.

Delirium: disorder of consciousness in which the patient is acutely disorientated, restless and confused. May also experience hallucinations and anxiety.

Delusion: a fixed belief which is held unshakeably and is out of keeping with the patient's cultural and social background.

Delusional perception: new and delusional significance is attached to a real perception without any logical reason.

Dependence: psychological and/or physical effect of habitual use of a drug/substance. Leads to compulsion to keep taking the drug. In physical dependence there are withdrawal symptoms if the drug is stopped. Psychological dependence means the person feels the need to keep taking it for well-being, but there are no physical withdrawal effects.

Depersonalisation: an unpleasant sensation where the person feels unreal or strangely altered, or feels that the mind has become separated from the body. Mild forms can occur in normal individuals under stress.

Depot medication: usually refers to long-acting injectable antipsychotics prescribed to patients due to a variety of clinical indications, including poor compliance.

Derealisation: a feeling of unreality in which the environment is experienced as unreal and as flat, dull or strange. Can be very frightening. Often occurs at the same time as depersonalisation.

Diurnal mood variation: variation in mood during the course of the day; usually low mood is worst in the morning.

Dizygotic twins: twins formed from fertilisation of two eggs. Share half the same genes. They are no more alike than siblings.

DSM-IV(*Diagnostic and Statistical Manual of Mental Disorders*, 4th edn.): published by the American Psychiatric Association and used in the USA (see ICD-10).

Dysphasia: disorder of language as a result of cortical damage affecting the generation and content of speech. *Aphasia* is a complete absence of speech due to cortical damage.

Dysthymia: chronic low mood not meeting requirements for a depressive episode.

Dystonia: postural disorder caused by disease of the basal ganglia. Spasms in the muscles of the shoulders, neck, trunk and limbs.

Echolalia: pathological repetition of the words spoken by another person.

Echopraxia: pathological imitation of the actions of another person.

EEG (electroencephalogram): measures the electrical activity of the brain. Reflects the state of the patient's brain and level of consciousness.

Elated mood: more cheerful than normal.

Erotomania: delusion that the individual is loved by some person, often a person of some importance.

Euphoria: exaggerated feeling of well-being.

Euthymia: normal mood.

Flight of ideas: speech consists of a stream of accelerated thoughts with abrupt changes from topic to topic. The connections between topics may be chance relationships, verbal associations, e.g. alliteration, but can usually be followed (unlike knight's move thinking). Associated with pressure of speech.

Formication: a somatic hallucination in which insects are felt to be crawling on/under skin.

Free association: articulation of all thoughts that come to mind.

Habituation training: training to decrease reaction and sensitivity to a fearful stimulus.

Hallucination: sensory experience in the absence of a stimulus. May be auditory, visual, olfactory, gustatory, tactile.

Hyperacusis: increased sensitivity to sounds.

Hyperaesthesia: sensations appear increased.

Hypoaesthesia: sensations appear decreased.

Hypochondriasis: fear of having a serious illness, in the absence of any real organic pathology.

ICD-10 (10th revision of the *International Classification of Diseases*): published by the World Health Organization, Geneva, 1992. Used in Europe for classification of mental disorders (see DSM-IV).

Illusion: false perception due to misinterpretation of a stimulus arising from an object.

Inappropriate affect: an affect that is inappropriate for the circumstances, e.g. giggling when talking about the death of a loved one.

Insight: degree of correct understanding the patient has of the condition and its cause, as well as their willingness to accept treatment.

Jamais vu: illusion of failure to recognise a familiar situation.

Knight's move thinking: odd, tangential associations between ideas leading to disruptions in speech, which means that the connections between topics cannot be followed (unlike flight of ideas).

Labile affect: affect repeatedly and rapidly shifts, e.g. anger to sadness.

Life events: psychologically stressful events in life (such as bereavement, divorce, moving house, changing jobs, etc.), which may trigger onset/relapse of psychiatric conditions.

Logoclonia: the last syllable of the last word is repeated.

Loosening of associations: the connections between a patient's thoughts are difficult to follow.

Monozygotic twins: twins resulting from fertilisation of a single egg. They have identical genes.

Mood: pervasive and sustained emotion that colours the person's perception of the world.

Multidisciplinary team (MDT): the whole team of mental health professionals taking care of a patient. May include psychiatrist, psychologist, nurses, social workers, occupational therapists, speech and language therapists, etc.

Mutism: total loss of speech.

Negativism: motiveless resistance to commands and attempts to be moved.

Neologism: a new word invented by the patient, usually with a personal meaning.

Obsession: intrusive or unwanted thought, image or idea, which enters the patient's consciousness despite attempts to suppress it.

Organic disorder: disorder due to change of structure of an organ or tissue.

Overvalued idea: unreasonable and sustained intense preoccupation maintained with less than delusional intensity.

Palilalia: a word is repeated with increasing frequency.

Passivity phenomenon: delusional belief that an external force is controlling aspects of the self, e.g. thoughts, impulses, actions.

Perseveration: mental operations, speech and behaviour carried on beyond the point at which they are appropriate.

Posturing: an inappropriate or bizarre bodily posture adopted continuously over a long period.

Poverty of speech: very reduced speech.

Pressure of speech: speech is very fast, as though there are too many ideas to verbalise all at one time. Occurs in mania and psychosis.

Prodrome: a symptom indicating the onset of a disease, e.g. strange feelings/aura before an epileptic fit, periods of depression before first schizophrenic episode.

Prosopagnosia: inability to recognise faces.

Pseudo-dementia: clinically similar to dementia but has a non-organic cause, e.g. depression, hypothyroidism.

Pseudo-hallucination: a form of imagery arising in the subjective mind, lacking the substantiality of normal perceptions.

Psychoactive substance: substance which acts on the brain to alter mood/state of arousal.

Psychomotor: muscular and mental activity. Muscular activities are affected by cerebral disturbance.

Psychomotor agitation: excess overactivity and restlessness, e.g. in agitated depression.

Psychomotor retardation: reduced muscular and mental activity. May occur in treatment with neuroleptics, but is characteristic of depression.

Puerperal: relating to childbirth or the period that immediately follows it.

Serotonin (also known as 5-hydroxytryptamine (5-HT)): a neurotransmitter thought to be reduced in depression. Also involved in sleep regulation.

Somatic passivity: delusional belief that one is a passive recipient of bodily sensations or movements from an external agency.

Somatic symptoms: relating to the body rather than the mind.

Stereotypy: repeated regular fixed pattern of movement or speech which is not goal directed.

Tardive dyskinesia: involuntary chewing or grimacing movements due to long-term treatment with neuroleptics.

Thought blocking: a sudden interruption in the train of thought occurs, leaving a blank after which what was being said cannot be recalled.

Thought broadcast: the belief that thoughts are audible to others or are being broadcast on television/radio.

Thought insertion: the belief that thoughts are being put into the mind by an external force.
Thought withdrawal: the belief that thoughts are being taken out of the mind by an external force.
Tics: repeated irregular movements involving a particular group of muscles.
Torticollis: the head is held constantly to one side.
Transference: the unconscious process in which emotions and attitudes experienced in the patient's childhood are transferred to the therapist.
Word salad: the speech is an incoherent and incomprehensible mix of words and phrases.